ADRENAL SYNDROME

The disease no doctor wants to treat

ADRENAL SYNDROME

The disease no doctor wants to treat

By G.E. Poesnecker, N.D., D.C.

G. E. Poesnecker, D.C. N.D.
Humanitarian Publishing Company
R.D. 3, Clymer Road
Quakertown, PA 18951

Library of Congress Card Catalog Number 83-080029

Foreword

"Creative insight" is the quality which is responsible for most major contributions to the field of medicine. Never "overlooking," always aware with a keen eye to observe and relate, Dr. Poesnecker exemplifies "creative insight" in its purest sense with regard to his observations of what he terms "Adrenal Syndrome."

Too often, complicated and varied symptom patterns are not given the thoughtful consideration that more common disorders receive. They are passed off as psychosomatic in origin or ignored therapeutically.

Dr. Poesnecker's insight led him to explore further just such a perplexing array of signs and symptoms, and reach a successful treatment regimen.

Contents

PREFACE

The Most Ubiquitous Disease in America Today

For over twenty-five years I have been studying a group of medical problems that have held at bay some of the best medical minds, both orthodox and unorthodox. Patients with these problems have been called neurasthenic, hypoglycemic, neurotic, psychotic, schizophrenic, paranoid, emotional, and sometimes just plain lazy. Their illnesses have been diagnosed as hyperinsulinism, hypocorticalism, anxiety neurosis, bored-housewife syndrome, hallucinations, depressions, obsessions, vitamin deficiencies, protein deficiencies, trace mineral deficiencies, cerebral allergies, food allergies, or something similar. Most of these patients have been treated for a specific diagnosed problem with some success, but only rarely have they been able to return to a really positive, functional state of health. The complete solution always seems to elude both the patient and the doctor.

In the past, much dedicated work has been done on many facets of this condition, and the individuals involved are to be highly commended for their efforts. Unfortunately, they usually presented their work as a specific disease entity, rather than as a part of the whole, which has given rise to the various terminology mentioned above. For this reason, patients with this problem often travel from one doctor to another, looking for help, only to have each physician tag them with his pet diagnosis, thereby creating more and more confusion in the minds of the sufferers who are already desperately confused and increasing the physical discomfort of the patients whose condition is not being treated.

With the publication of *It's Only Natural*, I released some of my concepts about these problems, and I feel it offered help to many patients who previously had found no real satisfaction (1). However, in the intervening years, new research has shed a great amount of light on this common and troublesome ailment. So much so that I hope at this time to present a truly comprehensive view of the condition and, for once, to bring the pieces of this complex puzzle together.

The most important reason for writing about Adrenal Syndrome is to attempt to reach the innumerable persons who have this condition but who are not receiving effective treatment. They are a great human resource going to waste. This book also is intended to serve as a guide and textbook for doctors who are aware of the condition but who would like more understanding on this subject. Patients who are undergoing treatment also can be helped to a better understanding of their condition by reading and rereading this work. Since these patients generally require constant reassurance, a book such as this can be extremely helpful.

A final reason for this book is not so easily stated, as it is based on my personal feeling. When a man devotes much time and energy to a project for the good of humanity, God blesses him with insight if his desire is strong enough. Such understanding carries with it a responsiblity for preservation. So, for what it is worth, I am moved to preserve the results of years of investigation and dedication to helping those with Adrenal Syndrome.

G. E. Poesnecker, N.D., D.C.

Clymer Health Clinic
Quakertown, Pennsylvania 18951

ADRENAL SYNDROME

The disease no doctor wants to treat

CHAPTER 1

The Nature of the Disease

Adrenal Syndrome is a condition of the neuroglandular mechanism of the body which produces a weakening in the body's ability to respond to stress. The most common symptoms produced by this condition are unexplained exhaustion, a tendency to be oversensitive and/or allergic to certain substances or environments, a lessening of the ability to reason rationally and to make decisions readily, a tendency toward low blood pressure, sensitivity to cold, poor circulation (cold hands and/or feet), and mental aberrations which can mimic a large variety of mental diseases. Most patients with Adrenal Syndrome have at least one of these symptoms, and some have all and many others besides.

This condition, to a lesser or greater degree, affects one-third to one-half of the American population. Luckily, most of those affected are not severely afflicted, but vast numbers of our people function at less than half their true potential because of Adrenal Syndrome. Since it is the nature of the Adrenal Syndrome patient to be a responsible, creative, and productive citizen, the loss to America created by Adrenal Syndrome is significant.

As common as this condition is, it is only indistinctly recognized and rarely treated by most professionals of the orthodox medical persuasion. For this reason, I call this condition the most ignored disease in the country today. Personally, I think this apathy has been produced by the general vagueness of this disease's character, by the neuroticlike symptoms of its victims, and by the slow and tortuous path of its correction even with the best and most advanced therapies. In our Clinic, I always meet the newly diagnosed hypo-adrenal patient with mixed feelings. I am, on one hand, pleased to know that the patient has started on the road to becoming useful and productive again instead of languishing in a low-functioning state; on the other hand, I always groan a bit inside when I think of the amount of care, time, and constant loving support that will be necessary to carry this patient through the seemingly unproductive early stages of treatment. With perseverance, however, all patients respond and, in the end, they prove to be among our most appreciative patients. This thought—at times, this thought alone—gives us the ability and the strength to carry on with the Adrenal Syndrome patient.

There seems to be a quirk in many doctors which, perhaps more than anything else, may explain their ostensibly conspiratorial refusal to recognize Adrenal Syndrome. Most physicians, in order to function as stable human beings, require a certain amount of personal ego satisfaction when they treat a patient. Even though there are vast fields of disease which are complete mysteries to modern medicine, the average day-to-day working physician often feels he must, at least in some manner, examine all the symptoms and problems that confront him. If he cannot rationally explain them, he must make up explanations and, if he cannot cure his patients, he must find some way to place the blame for his lack of understanding, knowledge, and ability on the patient or on the circumstances. In the early days of medicine, physicians had ready explanations for causes of symptoms and ailments which were presented to them. The fact that today we realize that most of these early explanations were ridiculous has not prevented the medical profession from continuing this practice. To witch doctors, all diseases are caused by demons which inhabit their patients. Their job, of course, is to extirpate these demons. The "scientific" physician, when confronted with a patient who displays the symptoms of Adrenal Syndrome, has a ready answer: "The patient is neurotic, mildly psychotic, unmotivated, or just bored with life." With that self-satisfied stance, that can be a "badge of our tribe," the patient is given a tranquilizer, antidepressant, or both and, with the fatherly advice to stop worrying and to go to work, he is sent home. It is just as impractical to tell a tubercular patient to go and play football as it is to tell an Adrenal Syndrome patient to stop worrying. Am I exaggerating? One has only to remember that a short time ago patients were literally bled to death in an effort to satisfy this medical ego.

There is, however, a specific cause that produces these wrecks of human society, and there are ways of returning these people to active, productive lives. This book defines this disease, lists the various symptoms produced by this condition, assesses the various stresses which trigger and aggravate this ailment, and outlines a comprehensive plan of treatment to overcome this insidious disorder.

The Adrenal Gland

Before proceeding with our discussion of Adrenal Syndrome, its causes and its treatment, let us consider the gland itself. The adrenals sit like a bishop's cap on top of each kidney; each weighs about a nickel. The adrenal gland is recognized as one of the body's most important endocrine or ductless glands, that is, glands that produce hormonal or hormone-like substances and discharge them directly into the bloodstream. Each of the endocrine glands is subject to a chain of command. The pituitary gland, so-called master gland of the body, sends out stimulatory or trophic hormones which regulate each of the target endocrine glands, such as the adrenals, the thyroid, or the reproductive glands. The pituitary in turn is regulated or controlled by the hypothalamus, which produces specific releasing factors for each of the pituitary trophic hormones.

The adrenal glands are composed of two parts—the medulla (inner portion) and the cortex (outer surrounding portion). The medulla fits inside the cortex like a walnut inside its shell. The medulla and cortex produce many substances, the most important of which are epinephrine (formerly called adrenalin), which is produced by the medulla, and various sterols, such as cortisone and aldosterone, produced by the cortex.

When the body is called upon to respond to stress, the adrenal gland is its primary agent. Stress on the body stimulates (probably by way of the sympathetic nervous system) the adrenal medulla to increase epinephrine production. This hormone increases the secretion of adrenocorticotrophin (ACTH) by the pituitary gland, which in turn activates the adrenal cortex to greater production of corticoids such as cortisone.

Diseases of the Adrenal Gland. Of primary concern in the discussion of Adrenal Syndrome is its differentiation from Addison's disease (organic adrenal insufficiency) and from adrenal insufficiency secondary to hypopituitarism. The term "Adrenal Syndrome," as used here, refers to a state of depletion of the adrenal glands in the *absence* of atrophy or destruction. In other words, it is a state of *functional* depletion or exhaustion. This is in contrast to Addison's disease in which there is physical atrophy or destruction of the adrenal glands, or to hypopituitarism in which there is some form and some degree of destruction of the pituitary gland. Both Addison's disease and hypopituitarism are relatively rare whereas Adrenal Syndrome, as herein described, is extremely common.

Diagnosis. At present, standard diagnosis of Adrenal Syndrome is a matter of exclusion; that is, such diagnosis is justified only after other causes of chronic fatigue, exhaustion, weakness, and lassitude have been ruled out. Unfortunately, the biological and biochemical changes which underlie this syndrome are poorly understood, and inasmuch as specific tests are not yet available, diagnosis depends on clinical features described elsewhere in this book.

Adrenal function may be assessed by standard laboratory tests which include serum cortisol levels and urinary corticosteroids. In Addison's disease, even in advanced adrenal destruction or atrophy, the resting or basal levels of these tests may be within the lower levels of normal. For this reason, a diagnosis of Addison's disease may depend on results of a pituitary stimulation test in which corticotropin (ACTH) is injected into the patient. In normal persons a significant rise in serum cortisols follows ACTH injection, but in Addison's disease there is minimal or no response. In cases in which pituitary insufficiency is suspected, the metyrapone stimulation test is utilized. These tests are described in detail in standard medical texts.

Standard medical texts state that clinical adrenal insufficiency (Addison's disease) usually does not occur unless at least 90 percent of the adrenal cortex has been destroyed by idiopathic atrophy, granulomatous destruction, or some other form of destructive process. By the same token, currently available tests, including the ACTH stimulation test, may not show abnormal results except in the case of advanced disease or depletion. On the basis of present information, it would appear that these tests lack the sensitivity to detect or diagnose lesser degrees of adrenocortical depletion, as in Adrenal Syndrome. Therefore, the condition of Adrenal Syndrome is largely undetected by orthodox measures.

History of the Disease

Early Recognition. In the past as in the present, there have been physicians who were not afraid to investigate the true nature of Adrenal Syndrome. The first truly clear-thinking researcher in this field was Charles E. de M. Sajous, M.D., LL.D., Sc.D. A Fellow of the American College of Physicians and of the American Philosophical Society, professor of therapeutics at Temple University in Philadelphia, professor at the Medico-Chirurgical College, and clinical lecturer at Jefferson Medical College, he produced a text in 1903 entitled *The Internal Secretions and the Practice of Medicine* (1).

In his book, he credited the physician, Brown-Sequard, as first bringing attention to the importance of the adrenal glands, in 1856. It was, however, through the experimental research work of Dr. Sajous himself, in our own town of Philadelphia, that the full significance of the adrenal mechanism, and particularly that part concerning the Adrenal Syndrome, was brought into full realization. In his book, he devoted an entire chapter to functional hypoadrenia much of which I include here, not with the assumption that all of its conclusions are accurate eighty years later, but to show the amount of knowledge accepted as standard medical information and procedure at that time.

According to Dr. Sajous,

> The adrenals playing so important a role in the maintenance of the life process itself, it is obvious that, apart from any organic lesion in these organs, any marked depression of their functional activity should manifest itself by symptoms corresponding with this depression. To the symptom-complex of this condition I have given the name of "functional hypoadrenia" to distinguish it from the forms due to destructive disorders of the adrenals, which constitute Addison's Disease and offer, of course, a far graver prognosis. As a definition of this condition, I would submit that "functional hypoadrenia" is the symptom-complex of deficient activity of the adrenals due to inadequate development, exhaustion by fatigue, senile degeneration, or any other factor which, without provoking organic lesions in the organs or their nerve-paths, is capable of reducing their secretory activity. Asthenia, sensitiveness to cold and cold extremities, hypotension, weak cardiac action and pulse, anorexia, anemia, slow metabolism, constipation, and psychasthenia are the main symptoms of this condition.
>
> The field covered by "functional hypoadrenia" is necessarily a vast one, since it includes the asthenias so often met within the four main stages of life: infancy, childhood, adulthood, and old age, usually attributed to a "weakness" or "exhaustion," and often "neurasthenia," which have been traced to no tangible cause. All I can submit herein, therefore, is a cursory analysis of the subject.

Hypoadrenia in Infancy and Childhood. In discussing functional hypoadrenia of infancy and childhood, Dr. Sajous pointed out that, although the adrenals at birth are one-third the size of the kidney and, therefore, relatively large, their functions are limited to the carrying on of the vital process, at least during the first year of life. During this time the mother's milk supplies the antitoxic products capable of protecting the infant against the destructive action of poisons. Dr. Sajous stressed the protective influence of mother's milk:

> It is an important function of the mother to transfer to the suckling, through her milk, immunizing bodies, and the infant's

> stomach has the capacity, which is afterwards lost, of absorbing these substances in active state. The relative richness of the suckling's blood in protective antibodies as contrasted with the artificially fed infant explains the greater freedom of the former from infectious disease.

He cited as striking proof of this immunizing function J.E. Winters' statement regarding the siege of Paris in 1870-1871 during the Franco-Prussian War: "While the general mortality was doubled, that of infants was lowered 40 percent, owing to mothers being driven to suckle their infants."

Children have a predilection to certain infectious diseases not only during infancy but through at least their first ten years. Dr. Sajous stated that mother's milk helps provide protection to the suckling against such diseases; vulnerability in older children is overcome as the adrenals, with other organs, acquire the power to supplant the mother in contributing antitoxic bodies to the blood. These facts, Dr. Sajous stressed, point to the adrenals and other prominent organs whose inadequate development explain the special vulnerability of children to certain infections. He believed that degrees of this hypoadrenia cause a child to be more or less liable to infection. He continued:

> That degrees of hypoadrenia exist in children is in reality a familiar fact to every physician when the signs of this condition are placed before him. The ruddy, warm, hard-muscled, heavy, out-of-door, romping child with keen appetite and normal functions, is one in whom the adrenals are as active as the development commensurate with its age will permit. He is ruddy and warm because oxidation and metabolism are perfect and the blood pressure sufficiently high to keep the peripheral tissues well filled with blood; his muscular, skeletal, cardiac, and vascular systems are strong because, in addition to being well-nourished, they are exercised and well-supplied with the adrenal secretion, which. . .sustains muscular tone. As normal outcome of this state, we have constant stimulation of the functional activity of the adrenals. The muscular exercise and maximum food intake involve a demand for increased metabolism and oxidation, and the resulting greater output of wastes imposes upon the adrenals, as participants in the oxidation and auto-protective processes, greater work, more active growth and development, *with increase of defensive efficiency* as normal result.
>
> The pale, emaciated, or pasty child with cold hands and feet, flabby muscles, whose appetite is capricious or deficient—the pampered house plant so often met among the rich—represents the converse of the healthful child described, just as does

> the ill-fed, perhaps overworked child of the slums. The emaciation, the cold extremities, indicate deficient oxidation, metabolism, and nutrition owing to the torpor of the adrenal functions; the pallor is mainly due to a deficiency of the adrenal principle in the blood and to the resulting low blood pressure, which entails retrocession of the blood from the surface. This child is not ill, but the hypoadrenia which prevails normally, owing to the undeveloped state of its adrenals, is abnormally low, and it is vulnerable to infection.

Sajous believed that all conditions which in the adult tend to produce functional hypoadrenia affect the child at least to the same extent.

Hypoadrenia in the Adult. Adults in whom adrenals may be inherently weak

> do not, as in hypothyroidia, show signs of myxedema; but their circulation and heart action are feeble, they tend to adiposis, and show other signs of hypoadrenia. I have witnessed suggestive bronze spots in such cases. As a rule, however, the development of the adrenals in adults is an accomplished fact—as also that of their co-workers in the immunizing process, the thyroid and pituitary. . . . The adrenals, fully capable of sustaining oxidation and metabolism up to highest standard in all organs, also preserve the efficiency of all other defensive resources, including phagocytosis, with which the body is endowed to their highest level. On the whole, the *normal adult whose adrenals functionate normally is relatively resistant to infection.* The infrequency with which the physician is infected, notwithstanding daily exposure in his professional work, attests to this fact.

Dr. Sajous explained that functional hypoadrenia appears when, irrespective of any disease, as the result of the vicissitudes of life, the adrenals are exhausted by excessive secretory activity that exaggerated labor or exercise—fatigue—imposes upon them. He cited a striking difference between patients with Addison's disease and those with other kinds of illness whose muscles are organically normal; signs of fatigue appear quickly and muscular impotence asserts itself in functional hypoadrenia patients but, for example, in an advanced case of tuberculosis the patient may be able to show appreciable muscular strength. He used other illustrations of the influence of adrenal secretion over muscular tone to show the close relationship between fatigue and the functions of the adrenals:

> The unusual prevalence of disease among soldiers in the field is, of course, partly due to the defective sanitation that a campaign

> entails; but fatigue—particularly that due to heavy marching, carrying heavy accoutrements—is, in my opinion, an important predisposing cause, through its influence upon the adrenals. Not only are these organs called upon to sustain general oxidation and metabolism at a rate exceeding by far that which amply suffices for normal avocations, but the fact that. . .they also serve to destroy the toxic products of muscular activity constitutes another cause of drain upon their secretory resources.

From studies of other investigators into the influence of fatigue on adrenal function in animals he noted that debility from any source—starvation, loss of blood, or other factors—makes the body vulnerable to disease. In a healthy animal, an injection of combined toxin and antitoxin resulted in no harm, but in an animal weakened by starvation or slight bleeding, death usually followed such an injection, with all the signs of poisoning by the toxin, including congested adrenals.

He pointed out the relationship between the adrenal gland and infection, adding that hypoadrenia from any source weakens the body so that it becomes vulnerable to disease. Among humans, he pointed to deficient food and excessive work as causes of the disease.

Other important morbid factors in this condition, according to Sajous, include masturbation and excessive venery. He wrote:

> The pallor and asthenia witnessed in these cases, so far unexplained, can readily be accounted for if, as I believe, the liquid portion of the semen is rich in adrenal principle. This is suggested by the fact that spermin, the purest of testicular preparations, given the same tests, acts precisely as does the adrenal principle. The latter is an oxidizing body acting catalytically; it resists all temperatures up to, and even, boiling; it is insoluble in ether and practically insoluble in absolute alcohol, and gives the guaiac, Florence, and other heamin tests. Now spermin not only raises the blood pressure, slows the heart and produces all other physicological effects peculiar to the adrenal principles, but its solubilities are the same; it gives the same tests; it resists boiling. Moreover, it is regarded in Europe as a powerful "oxidizing tonic" and has been found equally useful in disorders in which adrenal preparations had given good results. The inference that spermin consists mainly of the adrenal product suggests that it is not specific to the testes, but instead, a constituent of the blood at large; not only did this prove to be the case, but it was found in the blood of females as well as in that of males.

Hypoadrenia in the Aged. To Dr. Sajous, the ductless glands greatly influence old age. He wrote,

> all living organic matter is subjected, after more or less precarious periods of growth and adult existence, to one of decline and final disintegration. This applies particularly to the adrenals, if their functions are, as I hold, to sustain oxidation and metabolism, the fundamental process of the living state. Indeed, the senile state may be said to be as evident in these organs as it is in the features of the aged.

He quoted from investigators who had found that fat occurred in increasing quantities in the adrenal fibrous tissue between the cortex and medulla in very old animals and in the medulla of aged individuals. A marked—occasionally very great—reduction was found in the size of adrenals in the aged. In a study in which adrenals of three young men were compared with those of aged individuals, the adrenals in the young were well developed and in "full bloom," while in the aged they were shrunken and deficient, showing lowered activity, implying a lessening of the vital process the adrenal glands sustain.

"The asthenia of old age," he continued, "thus finds a normal explanation in the defective supply of adrenal secretion—precisely as it does in Addison's Disease. In fact. . .atrophy of the glands in the young may produce this disease." To Dr. Sajous, old age was caused by degeneration of the ductless glands. He believed that a condition of autointoxication existed in old age "quite in keeping with a decline in the antitoxic power shown by the adrenals." He also found a functional relationship between the adrenals and the thyroid in the genesis of old age.

Regarding the causation of old age, Sajous quoted an earlier researcher, Lorand: "It is evident. . .that all hygienic errors of diet or any kind of excess will bring about their own punishment, and that premature old age, or a shortened life, will be the result. In fact, it is mainly our fault if we become senile at 60 or 70, and die before 90 or 100."

As Seneca said, "Man does not die, he kills himself."

Summary of Sajous' Work. Sajous, then, believed that the lesions to which the adrenals are subjected during infections and autointoxication, from birth to the last day of life, greatly shorten life by limiting the functional area of the organs through the local fibrosis they entail. "It is quite probable," he wrote, "that centenarians owe their prolonged longevity mainly to integrity of their adrenals." To this end he saw hygiene, particularly its influence on the prevention of infectious disease, "as one of the most useful of sciences" because it helps prevent even seemingly benign diseases (diseases from which people recover), which "in the end shorten our existence by compromising the integrity of the organs which sustain the vital process itself."

Sajous discussed also the prophylaxis and treatment of the hypoadrenal condition. While much of the prophylaxis he discussed is not germane to the present day, he made several pertinent comments. In discussing prevention of hypoadrenia in infants, for example, he said:

> In infants, we should by every possible means prevent infection or intoxication to preserve the integrity of their adrenals and other autoprotective organs. The key of the whole situation lies in the fact that. . .nearly all the cases and nearly all the deaths are in bottle-fed babies. Physicians are, as a rule, entirely too ready to yield to the demands of social and other claims put forth by mothers who do not wish to nurse their offsprings. The responsibility assumed by both mother and physician under these circumstances is overlooked. I cannot but hope that if this continues, and the sacrifice of countless infants proceeds, laws may be enacted to prevent it by imposing upon the physician the duty of submitting to the State authorities a certificate in which sound reasons shall alone account for his consent to a departure from Nature's methods which entails deaths untold. . . .The death rate among foundlings in New York City reached almost 100 percent until wet nurses were provided. . . .Many. . .authorities have written forcibly upon this subject, but seemingly to no avail. The holocaust continues.

Dr. Sajous devoted several pages to proving that mother's milk contains antitoxic substances that are not present in the bottled variety. Surprisingly, only in the last few years has so-called modern medical science caught up with Dr. Sajous.

In referring to the prophylaxis and treatment of the adult patient, Sajous discussed the importance of rest, and of what physical stress with inadequate rest can do to the Adrenal Syndrome. This factor has changed little to this day.

> The influence of excessive fatigue on the adrenals, we have seen, is such as to weaken greatly their functional activity and, therefore, their oxygenizing and immunizing functions of the blood. The main harmful feature in this connection is the *relative* deficiency of rest, which means, from my viewpoint, inadequate opportunity afforded the adrenals to recuperate. This, of course, should be proportionate to the amount of strain imposed upon these organs, and the resistance of which they are capable. It is probably owing to lack of this that apparently strong men are often the first to "give out" in forced marches. The physical examination being

> based mainly upon the *status praesens*, and the adrenals being necessarily (for we are now dealing with a new line of thought) [Apparently still new today! — Author] overlooked as factors, there is marked inequality in the resistance of the men to strain. This applies as well to the pathogenesis of chronic disorders. In a personal analysis of 40 cases of hay fever, for instance, the severity of the disease corresponded to a considerable degree with the number of children's diseases the patient had had, the worst cases having had six of these diseases in comparatively quick succession.

To Dr. Sajous, this suggested the need of ascertaining the number and severity of children's and other diseases to which a recruit in the armed forces had been subjected and to add this factor to others in deciding upon his admission to the service or the arm to which he is to be assigned. He continued,

> The mounted man suffers less from actual fatigue than the infantry man who must carry his accoutrements, arms, cartridge, etc., aggregating in some armies as much as 70 pounds. When, besides, defective or poor food, impure water, exposure, etc., and other frequent accompaniments of a campaign are taken into account, one need not wonder that disease is a far greater factor as a cause of debility and death than wounds.
>
> Briefly, fatigue should be considered, owing to its inhibiting influence on the adrenals and the immunizing process in which they take part, as an important predisposing cause of disease. The periods of rest should be so adjusted, therefore, as to counteract this by far the most destructive factor of active warfare. In civil life, such hardships are seldom endured, but here likewise much could be done to prevent infection by means calculated to insure the functional integrity of the adrenals.
>
> To stimulate the adrenal functions when marked fatigue prevails would, of course, only aggravate the hypoadrenia after perhaps a period of temporary betterment. The powdered adrenal substance should, on the other hand, judging from the effects of injections of adrenal extracts in experimentally fatigued animals, serve a useful purpose.

In this last paragraph Dr. Sajous recommended taking powdered adrenal substance. To show that there is nothing necessarily new under the sun, this substance, properly prepared so as not to lose any of its natural factors, still remains the backbone of treatment of Adrenal Syndrome today. The work of this pioneering endocrinologist can never be sufficiently appreciated. We can only thank God for his great insight and candor, and attempt to carry forth the work he began.

Expanding Understanding of the Disease. A few years after Dr. Sajous' initial work, Henry R. Harrower, M.D., F.R.S.M. (London), in his book, *Practical Organic Therapy, The Internal Secretions and the General Practice*, asserted (2):

> Since the adrenals are so extremely susceptible to so many outside influences, it is likely that they would be easily worn out, and as a matter of fact, "functional hypoadrenia" is as common a condition as any endocrine manifestation. From a practical standpoint, this is an extremely important symptom complex.

This was written a short time after World War I! Dr. Harrower continued:

> It is quite some years since Sajous began to emphasize the importance of this condition, and while his opinions were scouted, and some of his ideas declared visionary, it must be admitted that our present knowledge of this subject is very much in harmony with the following quotation from Sajous' monumental work: "Functional hypoadrenia is the symptom-complex of deficient activity of the adrenals due to inadequate development, exhaustion by fatigue, senile degeneration, or any other factor which without provoking of organic lesions in the organs or their nerve paths, is capable of reducing their secretory activity. Asthenia, sensitiveness to cold and cold extremities, hypotension, weak cardiac action and pulse and anorexia, anemia, slow metabolism, constipation, psychoasthenia are the main symptoms of this condition."

Harrower went on to say:

> Asthenia is the rule and muscular tone (both striped and unstriped muscles) is poor. Exertion is impossible and the fatigue syndrome is prominent. The intestinal musculature is inactive and stasis, a common cause of hypoadrenalism, is also a usual result of it. Mental exertion, even the simplest exertion, often causes so much weariness and exhaustion as to be prohibitive. Mental elasticity is lost, and there is both mental and physical depression with the fear that the individuals now cannot accomplish their accustomed good mental work; and the story that they "have lost their nerve." With this, one frequently notes a fearfulness of making wrong decisions and vacillating and indecisive frame of mind. This is the most usual form of adrenal insufficiency. It is chronic both in origin and in its course.

Another section in Harrower's book is entitled "Neurasthenia as an Adrenal Syndrome." The word "neurasthenia" is not used as much today as it once was, nor is it as well understood by the general public as it was at one time. Neurasthenia means weak nerves. Although they may not have heard of neurasthenia, people frequently speak of their weak or sensitive nerves and upset nervous system. I personally still find neurasthenia an acceptable term and an exact description of many patients I see daily.

Again, Harrower's report was so lucid that I include here the entire section on "Neurasthenia as an Adrenal Syndrome":

> The minor form of "functional hypoadrenia" is more common than some have appreciated, and the fact that there is a psychic origin as well as the other physicologic causes already considered, allies it to the fashionable neurasthenia of today. In fact, some have stated that what is improperly called "neurasthenia" is not a disease per se, but really a symptom-complex of ductless glandular origin and that the adrenals are probably the most important factors in its causation. Campbell, Smith, Osborne, Williams, and others, including the writer, have directed attention to the importance of the adrenal origin of neurasthenia (though a pluriglandular dyscrasia is practically always discoverable), but so far this is not understood as well as its frequency and importance warrant.
>
> A few quotations from the literature will firmly establish the importance of this angle from which to study this common and annoying symptom-complex. Quoting from the *Journal of the A.M.A.* (Dec. 18, 1915): "The typical neurotic generally has, if not always, disturbance of the supradrenal glands on the side of insufficiency. The blood pressure in these neurasthenic patients is almost always low for the individuals and their circulation is poor. A vasomotor paralysis, often present, allows chillings, flushings, cold, or burning hands and feet, drowsiness when the patient is up, wakefulness on lying down and hence insomnia. There may be more or less tingling or numbness of the extremities."
>
> . . .Kinnier Wilson in. . ."The Clinical Importance of the Sympthetic Nervous System" makes the following pertinent remarks: "Many of the common symptoms of neurasthenia and hysteria are patiently of sympathetic origin. Who of us has not seen the typical irregular blotches appear on the skin of the neck and face as the neurasthenic patient works himself up into a state? The clammy hand, flushed or pallid features, dilated pupils, the innumerable paresthesias (tinglings), the unwonted sensations in head or body, are surely of sympathetic parentage. In not a few cases of neurasthenia, symptoms of this class are the chief or only manifestations of the disease. Here, then, is a condition of defective sympatheticotonus; may it not have been caused by impairment of function of the chromophil system [adrenal system]?. . .There does not appear to me any tenable distinction

> between the asthenia of Addison's Disease and the asthenia of neurasthenia. Cases of the former are not infrequently diagnosed as ordinary neurasthenia at first. It is difficult to avoid the conclusion that defect of glandular function is responsible for much of the clinical picture of neurasthenia. . . .[Wilson] makes the following apothegm: "Sympathetic tone is dependent on adrenal support, and until the glandular equilibrium is once more attained, sympathetic symptoms are likely to occur."

Interestingly, the 1915 quotation from the *Journal of the American Medical Association* postulated a relationship between neurasthenia and low adrenal function. Yet to this day, such a relationship is rarely considered in medical treatment. At the Clymer Health Clinic, we consider such cause and effect to be very common, and we treat it accordingly. Undoubtedly, because of this, we have become internationally known for our treatment of the weakened nervous system.

The most important advances in endocrinology made by Dr. Harrower were in connection with what he called the plural glandular treatment. In this form of treatment, he found it far more efficacious to use a variety of glandular substances than to use a single one in attempting to correct this or any of the glandular imbalances. In preparations he himself made and marketed, he, for instance, combined thyroid, pituitary, and sex-hormone substances along with what he called "remineralization" techniques; that is, the use of certain mineral elements plus his adrenal-gland substance to treat Adrenal Syndrome. Such plural glandular technique is used to this day. With modern methods of tissue-nutrition analysis, however, we are able to individualize the therapy for the specific case at hand to a far greater degree than was possible in Dr. Harrower's day.

While Dr. Sajous brought the condition of functional hypoadrenalism to light, described its symptoms, and some of its causes, and suggested certain types of therapy, the further development of this therapy was in the hands of Dr. Henry Harrower. Dr. Harrower's work, however, was little appreciated by his contemporaries and, although he was able to help thousands of individuals during his lifetime, he was never able to convince more than a handful of his medical colleagues of the value of the plural-glandular substance therapy. Since this therapy was based upon supporting nutritionally the glandular components of the body, the results, though definite and long-lasting, were slow in developing. This fact probably led the medical profession to disregard them in favor of the quicker-acting, but noncurative, single-hormone preparations and synthetic compounds.

It is important to make a distinction between the use of endocrine hormones and endocrine substances. Even these early investigators realized that if the body is given a hormone which is produced by an endocrine gland, the gland, due to the natural functioning of the body's homeostatic mechanism, will stop producing its own hormone as long as the external hormone is being supplied. If this process is carried out long enough, the gland involved will actually atrophy—eventually it stops producing hormones. If, on the other hand, a patient is given glandular substance which is free from hormones but contains the other nutrient elements of the gland intact, the substance acts as a food to build and regenerate the gland, so that it may once again start proper functioning on its own. This is the basic difference in theory and practice between the medical practice of endocrinology and the natural or nonmedical practice of endocrinology. These early researchers realized that, except in emergencies, nutritional glandular therapy was the only practical, physiological way of re-establishing normal function among the endocrine glands. In emergencies, it may be essential to give hormones in specific cases. Also, if the involved gland is destroyed, or there is no hope of regeneration, it may be necessary to give hormonal agents for life. However, in most chronic, glandular deficiencies, the use of glandular substance therapy is far more physiologically safe than the pure hormones.

Continuing Research. The work of Dr. Sajous and Dr. Harrower has been continued by a small group of medical practitioners, one of the most dynamic of whom is John W. Tintera, M.D. In 1955 Tintera reported on the hypoadrenocortical state and its management, and in 1966 he advanced the hypothesis that reactive hypoglycemia may result more from hypoadrenocorticism with deficient counter-regulatory responses of the adrenal cortex than from insulin excess (3,4). (A later study on hypoglycemia in insulin-dependent diabetic patients acknowledged indeed that deficiency in counterregulatory hormonal responses is important in hypoglycemia reactions [5]).

Tintera described, in lay terms, the functional insufficiency of the adrenal glands in an article in *Woman's Day* in February 1959, entitled "What You Should Know about Your Glands and Allergies" (6):

> Think of your adrenal glands as the two central command posts, one perched above each kidney from which your body's chemical defenses are mobilized and directed. Think of pollens, house dusts, and all other allergy-producing substances as attacking

> invaders (which they are, of course). Now you're right up against the basic and real reason why many people suffer from allergies while some people hardly know what the word means.
>
> What happens when the central command posts of allergic bodies fail to command the chemical defenders? Attacking invaders are on the ramparts, but the defenses are enfeebled and disorganized. The invaders get in and bring about the damage which results in wheezes and sneezes, sniffles, hives, rashes, skin eruptions, and other miseries and also sets the body up, chemically, for endless repetition of the same.
>
> This new knowledge discovered and proved by endocrinology, that branch of medical science devoted to the study of the body-regulating system of internally secreting glands, the endocrines, of which the adrenals are kings. Until endocrinology came up with the all-important knowledge, no one knew the basic cause of allergies.

Rightly, Dr. Tintera said that, until recently, there was no real, lasting cure for the allergies—only temporary relief which often required heroic measures. Usual treatments for allergies and infections were aimed at body chemistry disturbances at or near the surface.

> Actually, many allergies are only the end results of processes that have their beginnings in adrenal gland failure. Most people stand up well against attacking invaders—so well that they do not know they're under attack. But 17,500,000 Americans [almost 10 percent of the population] succumb so readily to the same invaders they know only too well they are being attacked!
>
> Endocrinology has now gotten deep down below the end results of allergy processes. In learning about the intricate and subtle chemistry of the adrenal glands, it discovered that the difference between the non-allergic majority was the difference between strong, alertly responsive adrenals which can and do marshal the body's defenses in a flash, and weak, sluggish glands which are incapable of doing what they should.
>
> I'm an endocrinologist. In more than 20 years of a busy practice with thousands of patients, I've yet to work with an allergic patient whose troubles weren't basically due to his poorly functioning adrenals, or who wasn't relieved of his allergic woes when his adrenals were put into proper working order. Included among these patients were sufferers of asthma as well as of hay fever, people "sensitive" to beef protein as well as those "sensitive" to house dust or to tomatoes or parsnips or whatever the so-called "sensitizing agent" happened to be.

To Tintera there are not "kinds" of allergies, only one "kind"—

impaired adrenal glands. For many years before this glandular basic cause was discovered, it was known that allergic persons were allergic to many—not just one—substances. He found the identity of the "sensitizing agents" of little more than academic interest because the controlling and only important matter is the state of the central command posts of bodily defenses, the adrenals. He continued:

> In understanding why this is so, let's begin with the fact that body chemistry is exceedingly intolerant of all substances not strictly its own. Foreign substances, for the most part, are broken down and converted chemically; animal proteins into human proteins, vegetable carbohydrates into human carbohydrates, etc.
>
> But there are many foreign substances which body chemistry can't handle by conversion. Some have to be neutralized chemically and so made harmless, and these are the "allergens" which cause allergies if neutralization doesn't come about. Others have to be killed or at least prevented from multiplying, and these are the living bacteria which cause infections if body chemistry fails to deal with them.

Taking ragweed pollen, for example, the pollen gets into the body through nostrils or mouth and burrows into nasal membranes. It cannot be dislodged by mucous flow or by sneezing, and it cannot be absorbed through conversion into a compatible chemical. If something isn't done, there will be inflammation and swelling of membranes of indefinite duration as more and more pollen gets in.

> So there is an emergency. The alarm runs along nerveways to the cores of the adrenals (the "medulla," in medical parlance). They respond by secreting a chemical or hormone. The blood carries it to heart, lungs, and other glands of the endocrine system, and back to the adrenal casings, the "cortex."...The medulla hormone stimulates lungs into providing added oxygen, heart into producing a faster blood flow, and the cortex into secreting a host of hormones which first call forth the neutralizing chemicals from various body cells, then put them together in assorted ways, and finally command their assault on the attacking invaders. All this happens in a flash. The amounts of chemicals involved are so very tiny they're hardly measurable. The increases in heart and lung actions are not enough for the mind to be aware of them. Just the same, a highly successful defensive operation has taken place. Definitely the body in which it happened is not allergic.

This defense, he asserted, takes place no matter where the attack occurs—in the membranes of the bronchial passages, the stomach lining, or the skin.

The principal defensive weapon on the battlefront of surface membrane is the "antibody." For successful defenses there must be antibodies for every variety of disease-causing bacteria or viruses; specific antibodies for pollen, for house dusts, tomatoes or parsnips, or whatever the foreign substance which is both inert and foreign and, therefore, is an "allergen."

The amazing thing is that the antibody for any given invader cannot exist until the invader actually attacks. Body chemistry takes the invader's chemical measurements, so to speak, and proceeds to tailor an antibody which fits the invader to a "T". This intricate, fast-moving chemistry takes place in the spaces between cells which are bathed in the body fluid called lymph. Lymph has chemical interchanges with the blood through the lymph channels and those channels have way stations or depots, the lymph nodes.

In the nodes, from materials fetched through the channels, are manufactured floating cells, lymphocytes, which first collect the newly-formed antibodies and then carry them to the membranes where the invaders, having caused the antibodies to be formed in the first place, are digging in. Now, we are at the key point. Antibodies cannot be formed and the lymphocytes cannot discharge their burdens of antibodies *without the assistance of the hormones of the adrenal cortex*. If the adrenal cortices are under-functioning, if they are semi-exhausted and unable to respond fully to stimulation, these essential hormones are either insufficient in amounts or they are chemically out of balance. Here, then, is the basic cause of allergies and infections.

Dr. Tintera explained that the cortex of the adrenal secretes no fewer than thirty-two hormones when functioning healthily. They and the hormones of the medulla are so vital in body chemistry that without them life is impossible.

Routinely they regulate the chemical conversion of our food into both fuel and building materials; they regulate the transport of the fuel throughout the body for "burning" with oxygen in each and every tissue, and the transport of the building materials and its uses in repairing and replacing old cells and tissues. On the emergency level, adrenal hormones prepare the body to withstand stress of whatever kind and degree.

Regarding stress, he wrote, "Walking is stress because it burns more body fuel. Running is a greater stress and so are heated arguments, tearful, and other powerful emotions, and thousands of other things which require changes in blood flow rate, in the diameters of arteries and veins, in the tensions of muscles."

All these stresses are perfectly normal and it is no less normal for our bodies to be under constant attack by "foreign" invaders since everything outside ourselves is foreign. But this constant attack is constant stress. Add everything together and you get the idea of how much work our adrenals are required to do. They are uncomplaining strong organs when all is well with them, *but some people are born with undersized or weak adrenals, due to the accidents of heredity.* (Emphasis added.) Under the stress and strains of living, the question for any individual is how much his adrenals can take; how much reserve strength. . .they have.

A person with very poor adrenals may never be affected by it if he lives a completely sheltered life, free of extraordinary stress. But that kind of life is neither desirable nor possible. Stress is the essence of living; from it comes pleasure and happiness. But if the adrenals are not thoroughly competent, each stressful incident cuts into their reserves. The day must come when those reserves are exhausted and the whole body is in trouble.

That explains why some people are allergic and susceptible to infections from birth while others are adults before those calamities befall them. One had poor adrenals from birth and the other had adrenals without enough reserves to last. And you can almost be positive that in any of these cases, the built-in weakness has been compounded many times by the common American diet which is bad enough to pull down even the strongest adrenals.

He explained that the adrenals in all his allergic patients are weak and semiexhausted, secreting their hormones in insufficient and unbalanced amounts. His treatment, to cure them of their allergies, is an injection of an extract of beef adrenals which contains the whole assortment of adrenal hormones in the balance drawn up by Nature. This permits the beaten-down glands of the patient to rest by adding hormones to body chemistry that take over the work. He does not use cortisone or its derivatives, except in emergencies, because, to be successful, the drug must be given in amounts that would upset the balances between the different groups mentioned and would cause adrenal atrophy if given over a protracted period. His patients were required

to follow a high-protein, medium-fat, and low-carbohydrate diet. It permits all meats and fish, all dairy products, all fruits, and all vegetables, except the very starchy ones. It forbids all stimulating drinks, especially alcoholic ones. It is the kind of diet that puts the least stress on the adrenals by permitting them to function with top efficiency, the kind of diet that does not exhaust but builds adrenal reserves. Fortunately, our adrenal glands have recuperative power; they will come back if given the chance.

We can see from Dr. Tintera's work that not only is the Adrenal

Syndrome problem flourishing at a later day, but it is actually much more pronounced than it was in the times of Sajous and Harrower. Why? Simple. Its causes are becoming more and more pronounced on all levels of our daily life with the continued assaults to our body by more and more sophisticated drugs and medicines and continued assaults from the outside due to increasing forms of pollution, contamination, and toxicity. The wonder is not that there are people who are affected by what I call Adrenal Syndrome; the real wonder is that there is anyone in the country who does not have this condition. It is amazing that any of us is able to function in an adequate manner and adapt to the great number of stresses and general assaults to the body that abound today. Dr. Tintera's work also reveals new aspects of the adrenal gland, particularly its control of allergies. Most patients who have allergies are victims of Adrenal Syndrome even though they do not as yet have the other classic symptoms. Dr. Tintera's comment on inherited adrenal weakness is also interesting. My work has consistently verified this point, and I now refer to these patients as having "Chronic Adrenal Syndrome."

Current Concepts. In more recent years relatively little has been done to explore and clarify the biochemical alterations in the body which cause Adrenal Syndrome. One research study, which reviewed the relationships between adrenocortical functions and infectious illness, stressed the presence of depressed adrenocortical secretion during chronic infection, although most information was based on studies of tuberculosis (7).

Perhaps the most exciting and promising advance toward understanding clinical disorders and illnesses brought about by early, delicate hormonal imbalances has been in the realm of thyroid physiology (8-12). This research has been concerned with relationships between hormonal secretions and depression. In studies of depressed patients testing with the hormones was the only early method of detecting hypothyroidism, as results of usual laboratory tests remained in the normal range. This research is exciting because revelations in this area may provide clues which will lead to better understanding of Adrenal Syndrome—not only its causes but the disease process as well.

Meanwhile, Dr. Hans Selye, the Canadian physiologist, in his long-term study of stress and its effect on the human body developed a theory which he called "General Adaptive Syndrome" (GAS) (13-14). According to Dr. Selye, the body contains a complex mechanism designed to permit it to adapt continually to the various stresses and pressures which assault it from all sides, inwardly and outwardly. As long as this system is capable of functioning in a more or less normal fashion, the human body and mind are able to adapt successfully to a wide range of stresses and assaults, whatever their nature—chemical, physical, bacteriological, viral, mental, or emotional.

Actually, this ability to adapt is common to all forms of life. When a life form can no longer adapt, it becomes extinct. In other words, this ability to adapt is the very essence of life itself. The mechanisms in the human body which produce this adaptation are, admittedly, complex and, as yet, not fully understood, but one of the most important entities in this adaptation is the adrenal gland. Without this small but mighty gland sitting like a bishop's cap on the top of the kidney, we would not be capable of adaptation. With a strong and vital adrenal gland, we are capable of adapting to almost everything Nature and life can throw at us. With a weakened or poorly functioning adrenal gland, the ability to adapt becomes more and more difficult until a point is reached at which it is difficult for an individual to function productively in our stress-filled, high-adaptability-requiring society.

Because of the central position of this gland in general adaptive syndrome, I call the condition, which basically is a poorly functioning ability to adapt, the Adrenal Syndrome. The name is short and descriptive, though certainly not all-inclusive. It should not be confused with other presently known conditions, except possibly Addison's disease; but, since this condition is caused by distinct pathology of the adrenal gland, differentiation should be easy. Henceforth, in this book, when I speak of Adrenal Syndrome, I refer to that condition of the neuroglandular system which produces a weakening or breakdown in the body's general adaptive mechanism.

The whole theory behind the Adrenal Syndrome can be stated simply if we take into consideration the previous discussion. There is within the body a mechanism which controls: 1) tissue repair and regeneration, 2) one's ability to fend off substances which might cause allergic or similar reactions in the body, 3) one's ability to withstand stress and to be capable of meeting the needs of the environment at any specific time, and 4) the mechanism to prevent or overcome all forms of disease. It is this system which animates and vitalizes us to become vibrant, useful members of society. As long as this system functions normally, there are few problems of life, be they physical, mental, or emotional, which we cannot overcome. It is the great productive center of all strength and vitality in the body. No matter what difficulties the body may encounter, as long as this adaptive mechanism is functioning well, we have every opportunity to overcome these problems. If there is a weakening or a breakdown in this system, everything else in life falters. Every molehill which the average person would leap with ease becomes an insurmountable mountain to the individual with Adrenal Syndrome. The simplest of life's tasks becomes complicated and monumental when the general adaptive mechanism is not up to par. At first the mind still functions and ambition is alive, but the body is not capable of carrying out the directions of these motivators. Eventually, frustration develops which causes depression, further exhaustion occurs due to stress and worry, and finally even ambition and mental capabilities themselves come under the influence of this weakened system. In extreme cases, suicide is not unknown among the victims of this disorder.

Causes of the Condition

What causes this system breakdown? Why are some people affected and others not? There are two common causes of this condition. They are often mixed in the sufferer to the point that it is difficult to say which actually caused the disorder in any specific case. The two causes are hereditary weakness and overwhelming stress. After twenty-five years of working with this condition, I feel that inherent hereditary weakness of the system is probably the most consistent cause of the difficulty. The glandular weakness seems to be passed down from one generation to another, the most common relationship being from mother to daughter, although any genetic combination is possible. Without adequate treatment, each succeeding generation becomes worse than the previous generation. Therefore, in most Adrenal Syndrome cases, the sufferer has inherited a lessened ability to adapt to the stresses of life. To make this more readily understandable to the patient, I usually refer to this situation as the inheritance of a weakened or poorly vascularized adrenal gland. While this is not entirely scientifically correct, there being other factors in a deficient general adaptive system, this is easy for the patient to comprehend and is not far from the truth.

Some persons' adaptive mechanisms are so weak that no matter how they govern their lives, they are destined to have a problem with this system. Such a problem usually begins at puberty from the stresses of the glandular changes which occur at this time. These patients come to us and say, "I've been tired as long as I can remember, Doctor. I never have had the energy or the ability to do what other people do with ease." The majority of hereditary adrenal cases, however, have sufficient adrenal functioning to live a relatively stable, normal life until a truly overwhelming continuing stress presents itself which exhausts the adaptive mechanism and finally throws these patients into full Adrenal Syndrome. These patients show the working of the two basic causes of Adrenal Syndrome: First, a hereditary weakness of the basic system itself; and, second, stresses of various types which are able to exhaust the functioning of the mechanism. The combination of these factors, however, varies tremendously in any specific case. For instance, as previously mentioned, it is possible for an individual to be born with such a weakened adaptive system that almost any of the normal adaptive needs of life can throw that person deeply into Adrenal Syndrome. Patients with this weakness are to be greatly pitied for, until they receive proper treatment, they never are able to experience the real pleasures and satisfactions of life. Then there are patients who have some weakness of the adrenal system but who can live fairly normally until the stresses in their lives start piling up, forcing them into the symptomatology of Adrenal Syndrome. Next, there are individuals who are blessed with a fairly normal adrenal mechanism, but who are unfortunate enough in life, as Shakespeare put it, "To suffer the slings and arrows of outrageous fortune," and to have stresses and pressures so enormous and so unresolved that the normal-functioning adrenal system with which they are blessed is no longer capable of sustaining their needs. It eventually weakens and plunges them into some variety of Adrenal Syndrome. Last, there are the fortunate persons whose adrenal or general adaptive mechanism is so strong that almost nothing in life can affect it. They are capable of going through all possible stresses and, therefore, they do not fall into Adrenal Syndrome, no matter what occurs.

Most of us fall somewhere in between the extremes of the last category of individuals who possess a strong general adaptive mechanism and the first-mentioned case of the unfortunate patients with serious hereditary inadequacy.

Almost all of us feel the effects of lowered adrenal functioning at some time in our lives, usually following a bacterial or viral infection or after some particularly grueling mental or emotional stress. At such a time, we often experience a temporary weakness and an inability to do our regular tasks as efficiently and as accurately as we would like. This is the result of adrenal exhaustion. If we are wise, at this time we will rest and not attempt to force ourselves to do more than our weakened ability readily allows. If we obtain sufficient sleep, stay on a healthful diet, and do not force ourselves to work until our strength returns, our adrenal system will shortly regenerate. The Adrenal Syndrome patient is constantly in a state that the average human being experiences only occasionally. In Chapter II of this book, "The Nature of the Adrenal Patient," this state is discussed at great length.

As can be seen from the above discussion, Adrenal Syndrome is due to a malfunctioning of the neuroglandular system of the body. It is caused by a breakdown in a physical component of the human system. Unfortunately, most of the symptoms which are produced lead the person to feel, from their vagueness, that the main difficulty is one of a mental or an emotional nature. The symptoms of Adrenal Syndrome are almost identical to those caused by anxiety and various other mental conditions. When we are fearful or in a state of depression, these emotional states cause various glandular mechanisms of the general adaptive system to produce secretions which cause symptoms similar to mental problems. Cold sweating, dry throat, rapid and irregular heartbeat, dizziness, cloudiness of the mind, nausea, flushing of various parts of the body, and so on, can all be caused by various emotional effects on the general adaptive system. These symptoms are the body's attempt to prepare us for a possible threat which does not exist, except in our fears. For instance, if we were out in the woods hunting, the cry of a wildcat behind us would create a certain sense of fear. This fear would cause the body to prepare for what is known as the "fight or flight" mechanism—either to fight this danger or to run away from it as rapidly as possible. When, in our modern life, we develop an emotional fear or apprehension, the body mechanism is not always capable of distinguishing it from a true danger; therefore, through the glandular system, it prepares us in the same manner as if we were ready to elude a real danger. Since there is no real danger and subsequent action, we do not readily utilize the hormones which were pumped into our systems, and thus a variety of symptoms are produced as these hormones first register and then slowly dissipate.

Many modern psychologists and psychiatrists recommend physical activity, such as running or jogging, to help allay the symptoms of anxiety and similar difficulties. What is occurring, of course, is that the various anxiety-produced substances are being more naturally utilized by the physical activity and are not left lying around, as it were, to create more physical symptoms to aggravate the original anxieties further. This therapy has much merit although it is not an answer to the original anxiety. In Adrenal Syndrome this same admixture, which is produced by the anxious patient, is produced by the weakened glandular system itself in an effort to bring its body hormone levels up to the normal level. Thus, we have a situation in which a person is not necessarily anxious or emotionally distraught and yet the physical weakness (the Adrenal Syndrome) produces symptom patterns which are almost identical to those produced in the nervous, neurotic individual. Just imagine what can happen to the patient suffering from this condition who goes to the average physician! Since there are no specific laboratory tests which identify Adrenal Syndrome in its earlier stages, the doctor finds no known disease process; and since the patient's symptoms mimic those of an emotional or mental difficulty, it is little wonder that the physician usually diagnoses the condition as mental anxiety. The patient is advised to stop worrying, told to go home and relax, given either a tranquilizer or antidepressant or both, and summarily dismissed. This is not meant as a criticism of the doctor who followed recommended medical therapy; in fact, almost any competent medical authority not conscious of or skilled in the diagnosis of Adrenal Syndrome would come to the same conclusion. Most Adrenal Syndrome patients are convinced by the time we see them that they are mental cases. They have been assured by their physicians, their friends, and even their loved ones that there is nothing wrong with them that a change of mind, a change of the way that they look at their lives, or a few tranquilizers won't help. This is not true. They are individuals with a true physical disorder as specific as if they had pneumonia or tuberculosis. You might as well tell the tubercular individual to stop coughing as to tell the Adrenal Syndrome patient to stop worrying or to stop feeling so tired and do an honest day's work like any normal human being. Persons afflicted with Adrenal Syndrome simply are not normal human beings; they are individuals with a real problem who need real treatment and real understanding.

An Ominous Triad

Thus, Adrenal Syndrome may be viewed as a triad, all three parts of which must be considered in every case: First, the heredity factor on which all prognosis or outcome is based. Second, the stress component which is composed of stresses that may cause the Adrenal Syndrome or be caused by it. Third, the group of symptoms which, due to the nature of the condition, are not only caused by the condition, but can become stresses which further aggravate the condition.

We therefore can amplify our original definition by stating that Adrenal Syndrome is that condition of the neuroglandular system which can be produced in an hereditarily weakened structure by a multitude of possible stresses which, in turn, cause a variety of symptom patterns which can in themselves become stresses, thus creating a self-perpetuating disease.

The whole condition sounds ominous and almost hopeless of resolution, and so it must seem to the afflicted patient. For it is a condition that not only can be triggered in sensitive people by ordinary stresses of life, but which actually produces its own stresses via its symptomatology. We might say it is a condition which feeds upon its own excrement. As we come to understand more about the character of this disease, we see why it is so neglected and so prevalent.

To understand it more fully and to become knowledgeable in its treatment, we must comprehend the interplay and ramifications of its three sides: heredity, stresses, and symptoms.

Heredity. Little can be done about the inherited factor except to attempt to determine its extent since all treatment and prognosis (length of treatment and chance of complete recovery) depend on this fact. If inherited weakness is great, treatment must be extensive and great efforts must be made to reduce all patient stresses to a minimum. Conversely, if the heredity factor seems slight, treatment and stress reduction can be much less stringent and a quick recovery can be assured.

There is unfortunately no simple, exact way to determine the degree of hereditary weakness in any specific case. A clinician with much experience can usually make a true estimate from the case history. Three matters are of prime importance: the age at which the symptoms began, the severity of the symptoms, and the amount of stress necessary to produce the symptoms. If the symptoms began early, were severe, and seemed to set in with no appreciable external stress, the heredity factor is strong and such a case will require the best therapy we have.

As a general guide, we can say that the degree of inherited neuroglandular weakness is in direct proportion to the severity of the patient's symptoms and inversely proportional to the stresses involved and the age at which they began.

Stress. Much has been written here concerning stress, but little has been written to define the stress; to understand the stresses that affect Adrenal Syndrome—not only that cause it but also that exacerbate it—is to understand the syndrome itself.

A stress in this context can be defined as any factor which stimulates the general adaptive system. These stresses can be divided into several types: First, those stresses which would affect all human beings somewhat alike, i.e., cold, heat, physical exertion, infectious diseases, toxic substances, malnutrition, and such things as exposure to war, flood, earthquake, and fire. Second, stresses which are individual due to personal background and experience. For instance, you may have a relative to whom you owe a large sum of money which you are unable to pay. Word of his return from a long journey may gladden the hearts of the rest of his family, but it can strike fear and consternation in yours because of the debt. This example of personal duress is the type of unseen stress that is usually the most difficult to diagnose and correct. Third, stresses which develop from the condition itself. The Adrenal Syndrome usually causes a weakened digestive function which, in turn, has an effect on the pancreas to produce a hypoglycemic condition which in turn produces more stress. This weakened digestion also allows many foods to enter the blood stream incompletely broken down, thereby stimulating the body to produce antibodies to attempt neutralization of the foreign substance. These antibodies, when they next contact this food substance, produce certain end products which may act as cerebral allergens, causing a variety of stress symptoms. These are only two of the stresses caused by this condition of the adaptive mechanism, but the list is long and readily shows the self-perpetuating nature of Adrenal Syndrome.

A full understanding of the stresses involved in Adrenal Syndrome is vital to recovery because all treatment is based on two simple principles on which the physician and the patient must work together. One, do all possible to build strength into the adaptive mechanism, and, two, remove as many stresses from this mechanism as possible. Unless the nature of the stresses are understood, they cannot be removed from a person's life. Some stress admittedly is useful, but long experience has taught me that no matter how hard a physician and a patient work, there will always be stresses left. It was Benjamin Franklin who said, "Those who have nothing to worry about will worry about nothing."

Symptomatology. Symptoms of Adrenal Syndrome are unique not so much because of their basic character, for these are symptoms common to other conditions, but because they themselves can have a profound effect on the course and progress of the disease. To understand this facet of Adrenal Syndrome, let us examine a typical patient. Let's take a working mother who is developing the condition and who of late has been experienceing unusual and unexplainable symptoms, such as strange tinglings, dizziness, mild nausea, the inability to concentrate, difficulty in remembering and in making decisions, being constantly and usually tired, digestive disturbances, apprehensions and anxieties which do not seem to have a basis in fact but which come sweeping over her for no apparent reason. Every little thing seems like a mountain to her, every cry of one of her children sounds like a screaming siren in her ear, every request of her husband seems like an unwarranted demand. Why would she not be anxious? Why would she not wonder if she is losing her sanity? Why would she not manifest all forms of worries and fears which, by their very nature, create further stresses which in turn worsen the Adrenal Syndrome, which creates more symptoms, and so on, ad infinitum.

Symptoms of Adrenal Syndrome produce a snowballing effect and, unless they are controlled, there is little hope of helping the patient. Once these symptoms begin, they are sufficient in themselves to continue the condition regardless of outside stresses.

Attempting to explain Adrenal Syndrome is like trying to explain the feelings of a new mother to a man. Words can only approximate the experience and perhaps only poorly at best. Just as mother love is not reducible to mere language, the sensations of Adrenal Syndrome cannot easily be described.

Summary

Adrenal Syndrome, a condition of the neuroglandular system, produces a weakening in the body's ability to respond to stress and, if not arrested, can lead to a breakdown of the body's ability to function. The condition is not easily diagnosed; in fact, diagnosis is usually a matter of exclusion. Although Adrenal Syndrome has been recognized for over eighty years, it has changed little in symptom pattern and in treatment required. At the turn of the century, Charles E. de M. Sajous, M.D., pioneered in the study and the treatment of adrenal gland malfunction, citing fatigue and other bodily abuses as major causative agents. He gave then the same or similar admonitions to patients as we do now in the Clymer Health Clinic. Although we may be able to refine his suggestions to make his admonitions more specific and sophisticated for a more rapid and complete recovery, the basis of treatment was outlined long ago by this intrepid pioneer. Henry H. Harrower, M.D., in the period following World War I made advances in treatment of adrenal malfunction, using what he called plural-glandular treatment—which is used to this very day at the Clymer Health Clinic. John W. Tintera, M.D., continued studying adrenal disease, especially the relationship of adrenal malfunction to allergens. Another doctor who made an important contribution to this subject is Hans Selye, Ph. D. He identified the general adaptive syndrome theory, describing it as the mechanism by which the body adapts to various stresses and pressures by controlling tissue repair and regeneration, fending off substances which might cause allergic or similar reactions, withstanding stress, being capable of meeting the needs of the environment at any time, and preventing or overcoming all forms of disease. In what we call Adrenal Syndrome, the general adaptive mechanism is unable to perform these functions. In Adrenal Syndrome, the malfunction of the adrenal gland results from a negative interaction of heredity, stress, and a combination of individual symptoms.

CHAPTER II

The Nature of the Patient

In my original work on the Adrenal Syndrome, I described the nature of the adrenal patient thusly (1):

> Bef/ore discussing the treatment of hypoadrenalism used at our clinic, let's consider the nature of the person who is most likely to develop this disorder and the manner in which it is produced. If I could describe the hypoadrenal patient in one single word, that word would be "sensitive". He is cognizant of all that is going on around him, and he feels an overconscientious sense of responsibility about those near and dear to him and even about the whole world. This person's nervous and glandular systems are delicately balanced; yet he is willing to take the cares of the world on his own shoulders.
>
> Such a nature is not sufficient alone to cause adrenal insufficiency. In my own estimation, a hereditary weakness of adrenal structure must be present. There are some persons who fit this description but who nevertheless have sufficient glandular vitality to avoid adrenal hypofunction. On the other hand, we do find persons who are by nature not perfectionists or inclined to drive themselves, yet suffer from this ailment. In these persons, it seems that the hereditary weakness is so strong that even a relatively normal amount of stress is sufficient to cause adrenal hypofunction.

Differences in Degree of Symptomatology

Not counting various external, physical, bacteriological, and chemical stresses, the two basic causes of Adrenal Syndrome are unremitting stress on an individual and the degree of hereditary weakness in the basic neuroglandular system on which the general adaptive mechanism depends. The Adrenal Syndrome patient is a combination of these two factors. These factors can be in any proportion and the variation in this proportion produces the different reactions shown by various Adrenal Syndrome patients. For instance, a patient may have only a mildly weakened general adaptive system, but be subjected to severe and unremitting stress in his life. If so, there is a good chance that eventually the general adaptive system will break down. This patient is an Adrenal Syndrome case and in need of treatment; however, the character and extent of his problem are different from that of the individual who has a severe hereditary or congenital weakness in his system and in whom seemingly insignificant stresses can produce severe Adrenal Syndrome difficulties. Both patients require treatment and much of the treatment is similar, but the emotional counseling and the general tenor of the psychological approaches to these two patients are entirely different.

The degree of symptomatology in a patient can often be calculated as a sum of these two factors. On a hypothetical scale of one to ten, taking one as normal and ten as severe, the first individual might have a two on the hereditary scale, but a nine on the stress scale. Together they total eleven. On the other hand, the second patient may have a two on the stress scale, but a nine on the hereditary scale. Together they also total eleven. The severity of symptoms in these two would be similar because of the eleven reading, but treatment would vary because of the different causes.

Obviously, the person who registers one on both scales has little problem. If a person rates a five on both scales, he approaches the area of symptoms. As patients display greater hereditary weakness and stress, say a seven on one scale and an eight on the other, they are going to have larger problems. In assessing the nature of the adrenal patient, these two interdependent factors which produce Adrenal Syndrome must be considered.

All Adrenal Syndrome patients are scored on these two scales for degree of hereditary weakness and degree of stress, and the doctor who treats them must ascertain their score on each scale as accurately as possible in order to prescribe the proper treatment so they may return to normal.

Adrenal Syndrome patients should be divided into two separate groups. First, that group which I stressed in my earlier work which, although they have certain hereditary weaknesses, are basically normal human beings who have been subjected to various stresses which have caused a definite, demonstrable change in their general adaptive systems. Second, those patients, and unfortunately their number is large, who have such defective general adaptive systems that the ordinary and mundane stresses of life leave them exhausted and incapable of coping. The latter patients require the most understanding and the best treatment we can give. They require the full understanding and cooperation of their families and friends. They generally require life-long treatment of one sort or another to help keep the general adaptive system in a reasonable form of functioning activity. There are no factors in their lives which can be ignored. There are no thought processes in their minds which do not affect for good or ill their basic problem, and, yes, their entire existences. It is really for this group of individuals that this book was written. The first type of Adrenal Syndrome patients can gain adequate information for their needs from my original text, but for those sufferers whom I now call "Chronic Adrenal Syndrome" patients, the first work was only an introduction. For them, a complete commitment on the part of themselves, their families, their friends, and their doctors is absolutely necessary for a proper resolution of their problem.

It is true, stress is not what happens to us but how we react to what happens to us. This statement must be qualified, however. When an Adrenal Syndrome patient has advanced to a certain stage in his condition, his mind, due to a variety of difficulties the two most important of which are lack of oxygen to the brain and cerebral allergies, cannot properly evaluate the stresses under which he is placed. The patient's mind simply is not capable of reasoning to the extent necessary to prevent further damage to the general adaptive system. It is necessary that patients in this condition be placed in an environment which is as stress-free as is possible and given proper treatment until improved cerebral activity allows them once again to be able to regulate and evaluate the stresses of their own environment. These patients, usually those with strong heredity factors, are so overwhelmed by common stresses that life in an ordinary household becomes almost untenable until some improvement in their condition is made. The nature of emotional stress in the individual with a weakened adrenal system can be so complex and so incomprehensive to the average person, that he often may seem mentally disturbed. No other group of people more exemplifies the truth of Benjamin Franklin's statement, "Those who have nothing to bother them will be bothered by nothing," than do those with Adrenal Syndrome.

With a weakened adrenal mechanism, the tiniest molehill becomes a Mount Everest. The slightest misconstrued remark becomes condemnation of a major magnitude. The most sedentary physical task is an insurmountable obstacle.

Example of Hypoadrenalism

Hypoadrenalism commonly occurs in a person who has cared for a loved one through a long, extended illness. Take, for instance, a woman whose husband developed cancer and was operated on unsuccessfully. Physicians gave up all hope, but the man had a sturdy constitution and lived on for a year or so before he finally succumbed. The family, not wealthy could not hire nurses and others to care for him, so his wife took care of him. She often was up day and night, watching out for his needs. The man she loved for many years gradually changed. Little by little he withered before her eyes. His emotional nature changed and he became a most difficult person with whom to live. There were times she wanted to scream at him, yet she knew that would not be kind or socially acceptable, so she held it in. She could not get her proper rest. She did not eat properly because she had lost her appetite. Instead she snacked on foods that did not supply her body with the vital elements she especially needed at the time. Her adrenal glands, the willing servants that they are, kept pouring out hormones to sustain her during the entire time. Unfortunately, they, like her, got little respite.

The unremitting and constant stress intensified. Although the glands can recuperate during sleep to some degree, her rest was less than normal and her glands had little time for their own regeneration. But they are valiant friends; they did not give in. They kept functioning and working well beyond their normal requirements.

Finally, death came to the husband. But stress was not over for the wife. She had to deal with the undertaker and then the lawyers. Then the government, inconsiderate relatives, and other people disturbed and even preyed on the recent widow.

During all this additional stress, her steadfast adrenal glands kept working their best to produce the substances she needed to keep going. Finally, she was able to rest. The undertaker, the relatives, the lawyers, and even the government were satisfied. At last she could relax. What about her adrenal glands? They were exhausted. They, too, demanded a well-earned rest. As soon as the stresses were removed and the adrenal glands were not needed to the extent they had been during heavy stress, their function slowed to enable regeneration for the preservation of the whole physical system. The widow suddenly felt tired and exhausted. Expectedly, she went into a period of depression and exhaustion.

Depending on the basic hereditary integrity of the adrenal glands, at this point she might or might not develop hypoadrenalism. If the glands were basically strong and healthy, she would be able to recuperate and pick up her life in a reasonable time. If the glands were inherently weak, she might develop hypoadrenalism. If the glands were weak, when they became so exhausted, even with the rest they were receiving, they might not be capable of regeneration to their normal state. They still were functioning, or the woman would die, but at a level far lower than before the prolonged period of stress, much lower than the level needed for normal daily existence.

We have just reproduced a classic case of functional hypoadrenalism. Although there are many other ways of describing this syndrome, from this case history certain specifics can be derived about the nature of the stress most likely to produce this condition.

First, although the stress itself is not necessarily great, it is generally unremitting. Also, we sensitive humans are not able to overcome it—either because of a sense of responsibility or because of our emotional dependency. That is, even though it was exhausting her adrenal glands, the wife in the above example had no choice but to take care of her husband. For her own physical well-being, she could have abandoned him, turned him over to relatives, if such existed, or tried to get the state to take care of him. It would have prevented her from developing hypoadrenalism, but her own sense of responsibility would not have allowed it. In my experience, I have found most stresses that produce hypoadrenalism come from doing what a person believes to be his duty. If we are to prevent hypoadrenalism in those who are susceptible, we must teach them to learn to control their response to the stress.

Our attitude—what I call acceptance of the stress—is often on par with or even more important than the stress itself in producing reaction. For example, had the woman whose husband was dying been able to rearrange her life, much of her later trouble could have been prevented. She could have eaten foods and nutrients that are best able to build up the adrenal glands, supporting the glands through this difficult period. With more knowledge she could have changed her basic attitude toward her husband at this time to a complete acceptance of his condition and of his unavoidable death.

From the foregoing, one can readily see how easy it is to develop Adrenal Syndrome. The situation described is all too common, but the patient should be capable of responding within a fairly short time if she is receptive and if adequate treatment is given. The problem with so many cases is that only rarely is treatment given toward rebuilding the general adaptive system. The patient is usually untreated and must live through the ensuing years as best she can. Much of her ability to improve depends on the stresses placed upon her and upon the basic integrity of her general adaptive system. If her future stresses are within reason, and her adaptive system relatively normal, she may gradually return to a normal state of health and productivity, time and rest being a good doctor in this instance. On the other hand, if her adaptive system is marginal and the stresses of widowhood difficult, without specific treatment she may never return to normal and may even continue to deteriorate with time. If such patients would seek the help of professionals trained to intervene in this condition, much misery and nonproductiveness could be prevented. It would be interesting to take a survey to find out how many on our ever growing state and federal welfare rolls are actually victims of this disorder. The normal mind and body is a productive mechanism. It is designed as such and likes to work as such. When it does not, one certainly has the right to wonder if it is functioning normally or whether it is in some unknown manner defective. Are the so-called poor really lazy and hereditarily unproductive or are they perhaps victims in many cases of a dysfunctioning adaptive system?

Chronic Adrenal Syndrome

How do individuals with Chronic Adrenal Syndrome differ from patients with the simpler type? How can you as a husband tell if your wife has this problem? How can you as a mother tell if your son or daughter is a Chronic Adrenal Syndrome sufferer? How can you as a lover tell if your future mate may have this difficulty? The answers are not easy, but there are answers.

Differences in Types of Adrenal Syndrome. When I first interview a patient, I look into his eyes. The Bible says that the eyes are the windows of the soul. That may be true, but they are also the windows of the general adaptive system. Persons with Chronic Adrenal Syndrome show to a lesser or greater degree an appearance in the eyes that is unmistakable to the trained observer. They have a certain vague staring, a vacantness which in my experience is without precedent in other disease conditions. It is nearly impossible to describe, but the person who has seen it once will never miss it again. A similar appearance is found in those who are taking street drugs and in some who imbibe too much alcohol, but, while similar, there is a distinct difference between the look of the Chronic Adrenal Syndrome patient and those who have been taking drugs or alcohol.

When these patients are examined, a difference in their blood pressure levels between the reclining and the standing positions is often registered. In general, the blood pressure is somewhat lower than normal in these patients and tends to drop or at least not to rise as it should in the normal individual when they stand up from a reclining position. For instance, if a normal blood pressure reading is 120 over 80, Chronic Adrenal Syndrome patients may have a blood pressure reading of 110 over 70 in the reclining position, but when they stand, it may drop to 100 over 70 or even to 90 over 70. The amount of the drop is usually indicative of the severity of the condition. There are many qualifications concerning this testing mechanism, however. If a patient with Chronic Adrenal Syndrome constantly attempts to force himself to activity, he may show the same rising of blood pressures when he stands up as do normal individuals. However, after waiting a minute or so, the blood pressures will gradually start to drop because his adrenals are simply not strong enough to hold the higher level for any length of time. In my earlier book, I stated that the amount of drop in the postural blood pressure is indicative of the condition of the adrenal patient. This is still true, but, as suggested here, must be interpreted with many reservations. One has to know how to read these pressures and equate them with the nature and the state of the patient at the time of the reading. Of recent years I have come to use the expression of the eyes as far more indicative of the state of these chronic adrenal individuals than the postural blood pressure readings, although the latter are still of great value, especially if they include the resting pressure, the pressure immediately upon standing, and the pressure at 20-second intervals for a minute to a minute and a half while the patient remains standing. The amount of drop and the speed of drop as time progresses gives a good indication of the state of adrenal functioning.

In regard to postural blood pressures, a patient may come in feeling exhausted and yet have a good blood pressure reading. On the other hand, a patient may come in feeling quite well with a poor blood pressure reading. This may be explained by the fact that there is always a certain time lag between the exhaustion of the glands and the symptoms produced; blood pressure usually predicts how patients are going to feel rather than how they are feeling at that time. For instance, if a patient who is feeling poorly has a good pressure reading, I can usually predict with confidence that he will improve within a day or two and feel much better. On the other hand, if a patient feels good but has a poor reading, I usually advise that patient to increase his medication and to take it easy for the next few days or he will go into a period of decline.

Further information necessary to diagnose the Chronic Adrenal Syndrome case must come from the patient history. This history usually shows that the adrenal patient has had spells of exhaustion, weakness, inability to concentrate, poor memory, allergic sensitivities, sensitiveness to many ordinary situations, and so on, as far back as he can remember. Most often these victims started to notice their difficulties at puberty, although many assure me that they had the symptoms even earlier. There is a group which did not notice difficulties at puberty, but did notice them in their late high school years or when they tried to keep up with the rest of the students in college. In this latter group, most went away to college, lived in a dormitory or apartment, did not get sufficient sleep, ate poorly—either insufficient amounts or junk foods or both, had stressful relationships with members of the opposite sex, may or may not have had financial difficulties, and were overconscientious in their studies, often attempting to obtain grades which were beyond their native abilities. These stresses are exactly the type to trigger a latent Chronic Adrenal Syndrome.

Other histories show that the first signs of this syndrome occurred shortly after marriage or after the births of children. All of these events have this in common: They are normal stresses of existence which occur at various times in our lives and which our adaptive mechanism should take in stride, but which are sufficiently stressful in individuals with a weak adaptive system to trigger the full Chronic Adrenal Syndrome. This hereditary weakness must be compared to an internal bomb that only requires sufficient stress to act as the spark to light the fuse, and once it is set off, their systems, like Humpty-Dumpty, are difficult to put back together again.

The character and mechanism of a chronic adrenal case can generally be differentiated from the hyperstress-type case because the chronic patient shows symptoms at an earlier age, though not invariable so, but, more importantly, tends to be triggered by stresses which the average person should be able to handle without real difficulty. This last factor is the true dividing line between these two types of Adrenal Syndrome patients.

Symptoms Similar to Mental Illness. Most Chronic Adrenal Syndrome patients are considered by their friends, relatives, and health practitioners—the people from whom they seek aid—to be suffering from some form of mental or psychological disturbance. This is true to such an extent that during our first interview with them, the majority of these patients assert they are sure that they have mental or psychological problems. One of the first and most important tasks of our therapy is to convince them that this is not true. Unless we accomplish this, treatment is difficult and sometimes nearly impossible. Many of these patients are called schizophrenic, some paranoiac, some manic-depressive, and most are called neurotic. This is not to say that all schizophrenic, manic-depressive, or paranoid patients are Chronic Adrenal Syndrome victims. There are true paranoids, true schizophrenic patients, and true manic-depressives, but Chronic Adrenal Syndrome can mimic the symptom patterns of all of these mental conditions. What I am saying is that any person, who has been diagnosed as having one of these conditions, should be examined to also determine whether, possibly, his condition is Chronic Adrenal Syndrome. Such patients are brought almost daily to our Clinic. Many are helped because, as it turns out, they are suffering from Chronic Adrenal Syndrome and, therefore, can be treated by specific physical means.

Determining Characteristics. Having treated these patients for over twenty-five years, I have found a variety of interesting characteristics which are of great help in understanding and diagnosing these patients. A history of these might be helpful to those who are, themselves, wondering whether they or one of their loved ones might have this ambiguous but disabling disorder.

"Don't Make Me Wait!" It is difficult for these people to wait calmly for any length of time. Usually either one of two things happens when they attempt to wait. Either they gradually become more and more exhausted until they simply have to lie down and rest, or they gradually grow irritable to the point that they become extremely disagreeable, ready to lash out at almost anybody about anything. In our Clinic, I specifically tell all chronic adrenal patients that when they have to wait and feel either of these symptoms starting to come upon them, they are to let the nurse know that they can no longer wait and go to rest or enter some activity to relieve their anxiety. We then call them when a treatment room is available.

When an adrenal patient starts to feel this type of anxiety, he must take action, i.e., remove himself from the environment which is causing the anxiety, no matter where he may be. To sit and fight these sensations is to create more stress and tension, and, what is worse, this inaction can produce a destructive, martyred attitude. He might think: "Why does the doctor make ME wait?? If he is truly concerned about me, he would not make me sit here; poor little me." This attitude is common and understandable in Adrenal Syndrome patients, but it is unproductive and generally unfounded. These patients need only the freedom and the good sense to excuse themselves and to go somewhere to rest whenever this exhaustive irritation overcomes them.

Sometimes if I am not specifically sure of the diagnosis of a difficult case, I may let the patient sit in my waiting room for some time, observing him repeatedly out of the corner of my eye for signs and symptoms of either of these states. If either of these patterns occurs, I can be pretty sure that a diagnosis of Chronic Adrenal Syndrome is accurate.

"You Make Me Mad!" One somewhat common experience of these patients that had me befuddled for a while was finally clarified in my own mind by a clinic case. The patient, the wife of a judge in a southwestern state, was an obvious Chronic Adrenal Syndrome victim who had been placed on heavy doses of amphetamines for many years to keep her functioning. Even with these, however, she awakened in the morning feeling so exhausted and depressed that she had little desire to get up or to attempt any activity of the day. She had discovered, however, in some accidental way, that if she became angry, gradually she would start feeling better and eventually be able to get up and go about her daily duties. While she was staying at our Clinic, she vented her imaginary wrath on the first person she saw in the morning. This was usually a member of the kitchen staff bringing her breakfast. This anger was quite vehement, as extreme emotion was necessary to stimulate her poor, abused adrenals to even a modicum of activity. Of course, this daily occurrence was soon reported to me. Whenever I visited this patient a little later in the morning, she always was in a very pleasant and good humor as the wrath had dissipated as soon as the adrenals were stimulated. I could not understand about what the kitchen staff had complained. Only later, after the patient had left our Clinic, was I able to consider the situation calmly and understand the mechanism behind her early-morning tirades. In this particular instance, the taking of amphetamines for a long period of time had created such a constant stimulus to the adrenal system that even they were no longer adequate to get her glands started after a night's rest. It took the strong stimulus of rage to wake up her poor, weakened adrenal mechanism. The problem with this method of adrenal stimulation was that the degree of rage necessary to get her going

created severe stress on everyone around her. While this patient was at our Clinic, our staff absorbed the force of her conduct, but when she returned home, her husband was the sole recipient. Little wonder that he was anxious to have her remain with us!

While this was certainly the most extreme case we encountered of anger being used to activate the system of a chronic adrenal patient, this same action occurs to a lesser degree in many victims of this disorder. I have as patients many women with this problem who, when the stresses get too great, throw themselves into a state of severe hysteria and remain in this state until they have sufficiently stimulated their adrenal system and poured sufficient hormones into their bloodstream.

"But I Can't Forget It!" Another common characteristic of Chronic Adrenal Syndrome is the patient's inability to clear the memory of consciousness of personal problems so that treatment and cure can proceed. Probably because of poor circulation and, therefore, poor oxygenation that is common to the brain of these patients, the normal reasoning faculties, particularly those used to distinguish between that which is rational and that which is not, do not function as they should. Therefore, these patients have difficulty clearing their minds of certain thought processes which unfortunately remain imbedded, as it were, in the memory and constantly act as recurring stresses which make treatment most difficult. Possibly some specific form of chemical activity due to a failure of the general adaptive system allows this to occur in the brain. In the near future we may be able to ascertain this chemical activity and, by neutralizing it, hasten the patient's ability to free himself from these retained, unproductive thought patterns.[1]

A few simple examples illustrate this point. In an unguarded moment, a husband may have said something to a wife that she misunderstood and he did not fully mean. The normal wife can rationalize after a while from his actions that he really did not mean what he said and then forget it. The Chronic Adrenal Syndrome patient often cannot free the incident from her consciousness. She constantly turns it over and over in her mind, building stress to the point that she cannot sleep, and at times may go into fits of uncontrolled anger and hysteria. Counseling, even by the best of physicians, often has little effect on these patients. About the only help at the present time for this patient is an active treatment of the general adaptive system to improve the oxygen-

[1]A test to accomplish this, at least in part, may have been found. See the discussion of the X-K Test in Chapter VII, page 143.

carrying power to the tissues of the brain so that it can again function in a more rational manner. This will usually work, although it takes time to clear some patients' minds and the unfortunate obsession can be very painful and trying to those who are near and dear to these patients.

Or, for example, because of a patient's gradual deterioration into Chronic Adrenal Syndrome her husband may no longer think of her as desirable. He wants a divorce. She is told that the only way of preventing this is to once again make herself desirable. The way that this must be done is to cure her Chronic Adrenal Syndrome. However, the fear of losing her husband becomes such a chronic stress that it makes therapy difficult. As rapidly as treatment strengthens her general adaptive mechanism, she tears it down by worry and concern over a situation which can only be corrected by the treatment which she is negating by her actions.

Both of these cases illustrate what I mean when I say that this condition is self-perpetuating and malignant in its nature. It produces emotional patterns which, by their nature, tend to worsen the condition itself. These states I have called the "dead-end canyons of emotions," in that while the emotion exists, it creates nothing productive. All it can do is to tear down and destroy the basic functioning of the body.

These patients have a condition which is basically a general adaptive system weakness. Their bodies cannot adapt to the stresses placed upon them. In one group of patients, the body may be basically normal, but the stresses placed upon it are of such a magnitude that it starts to malfunction, at least temporarily. Treatment usually corrects these cases fairly quickly, and as long as the patients are somewhat careful of future stresses, they can usually avoid returning to the Adrenal Syndrome.

For the vast number of people who have an inherent hereditary weakness of this adaptive mechanism, knowledgeable and extensive treatment is usually required over a long period of time, but they can be returned to life as functioning, productive members of society. To achieve this end takes true understanding on the part of their physicians, their families, and their friends, and, to some degree, from society as a whole.

Relationships with Others

Mother-Daughter Relationship. Most Adrenal Syndrome patients show a strong hereditary influence which usually can be directly related to one parent or the other. The most common relationship that I have found is the mother-daughter inheritance. A woman who has an Adrenal Syndrome problem may have sons who exhibit the problem, but almost inevitably her daughters have Adrenal Syndrome. Conversely, when I see a young woman with Adrenal Syndrome, inevitably, on checking, I find that her mother has or had a similar problem.

The inheritance may come through the father and may, as mentioned, affect male offspring. But the invariableness of the mother-daughter inheritance is worth mentioning here. When we encounter an Adrenal Syndrome patient, we also make an effort to influence other members of the family to be checked for the condition. This is of great importance should a young mother exhibit the syndrome. While her children may be too young to show symptoms, we know from experience that unless their neuroglandular mechanisms are strengthened, they will undoubtedly have trouble as they approach puberty. In these instances, we try to institute minimal basic treatment at an early age to forestall the nearly assured development of Adrenal Syndrome in these young children. This is particularly important in the case of daughters.

Relationships that Strengthen or Weaken. Certain types of individuals help to strengthen adrenal patients, and certain types tend to weaken them. This susceptibility to individuals may vary greatly, depending on the state of health of the adrenal patient. Much of this has to do with the personality of the friend. Full of animal magnetism, some people have a surplus of energy and goodwill. The Chronic Adrenal Syndrome patient absorbs from these persons and benefits thereby. But the relative or friend must be careful not to let the adrenal patient absorb so much energy that he—the relative or friend—is left depleted.

Some people are "emotional vampires," so devoid of energy and love within themselves that they attempt to sap others whenever possible. If an Adrenal Syndrome patient gets into the clutches of one of these individuals, he can be drained of his remaining vitality in short order. In general, if a patient feels stronger after being with a person, well and good. But if the patient always feels worse, beware, for that person might be an enervating entity, an emotional vampire.

Those with a predeliction to Chronic Adrenal Syndrome seemingly by a natural selective process, usually marry an individual who is at the opposite pole of neuroglandular integrity—which is a scientific way of saying that a woman, who is delicate and weak in the neuroglandular system by nature, invariably marries a man who is strong and solid in his neuroglandular makeup. It is almost as if when she was young she knew that it would take a man of such qualities to watch over and protect her through the difficulties possible in the ensuing years. Often these individuals have little in common, but in the long run they need one another to fulfill specific purposes in their lives and so the marriages are generally successful, at least as far as permanence is concerned. I have known a few Adrenal Syndrome patients who married one another. The results were usually disastrous because of the instability of the chronic adrenal individual. Somewhere in their lives there has to be a rock-stable person to offer support and sustenance or their whole existence is placed on shifting sands.

An individual with Adrenal Syndrome can often help another patient, especially in the early stages, by letting him know that he is not alone with his unfortunate problem. One of the most common symptoms of the Chronic Adrenal Syndrome patient is a feeling that he has something which no one can understand and which no one has had before. Friends and relatives assure him that they have never heard of anything like it. This is, of course, because so few doctors acknowledge the condition and so little publicity has been given to it.

Mixed Vibrations. Many individuals who are drained of energy by those around them feel that they are victims of agoraphobia, that is, fear of crowds, mainly because when they are in a crowd, they find that they grow weak and anxious. Generally, this is not true agoraphobia, but merely the draining effect or what I call the "leeching effect" that crowds have on Adrenal Syndrome patients. This is one of the earliest symptom patterns I usually notice in Adrenal Syndrome cases. Years ago when I first started to practice in Seattle, Washington, a patient who had been a life-long music lover stated that within the last year she had enjoyed concerts less and less. It seemed that each time she went to a concert, she became exhausted and quite agitated. Upon examination, she was found to have a relatively mild adrenal weakness and, with proper therapy, was able to regain her health soon and fully enjoy her love of music once again.

Many Adrenal Syndrome patients are sensitive to the mixed vibrations of any large group of people. Each human being is a radio transmitter sending out a vast number of different frequencies which create a so-called "aura" or eminence about him. With most of us, our own vibrations are so strong that those of other people around us have only a minimal effect. To the truly sensitive hypoadrenal victim, however, this effect can be powerful, even to the point of leeching his very energy. His own vibrations can be so weak that he readily absorbs the vibrations and emanations which come from other people. Because of this effect, Adrenal Syndrome patients must be careful with whom they associate. On one hand, they find that association with certain persons tends to strengthen them as long as the liaison is not too long. On the other hand, they discover others who enervate them after a longer or shorter period. It is essential to their progress that they shun individuals who sap their energies. But it is to their benefit to associate with persons with whom they feel an increase in energy.

As the number of persons the Adrenal Syndrome patient encounters in a group increases, the chance of benefiting from the association decreases. As the vibrations of more and more persons are present in the atmosphere around the Adrenal Syndrome patient, the chances become increasingly great that the mixture of these electromagnetic vibrations will adversely affect the patient. Due to this fact, we usually recommend that these patients stay away from crowds as much as possible.

If there is a function the Adrenal Syndrome patient wishes to or must attend, however, we suggest that he remain for as short a time as possible, and, even then, try to choose such associations as carefully as possible to ensure many beneficial vibrations present. For instance, a patient may wish to go to a concert of classical music, and, if it is not too long, the patient may gain from the exposure.

Even Happiness Hurts. One characteristic of the neuroglandular exhaustion produced by Adrenal Syndrome that is different from the type of exhaustion produced by any other condition is that even events and circumstances which the patient enjoys or which might be a happy surprise fatigue and weaken him. For the patient who loved the chamber music concerts they were a great joy, and yet they created sufficient stress, because of the people involved, to be detrimental to her neuroglandular system. Almost all other forms of depression, anxiety, tension, and so on are improved by happiness and pleasant events. A surprise birthday party, a visit from a long-forgotten friend, or a telephone call from a sweetheart—all of these things strengthen the body and spirit of almost everyone except the Adrenal Syndrome patient. This is perhaps the saddest component of the entire condition, but it is nevertheless pathognomonic of the disease.

When an individual becomes exhausted or physically weakened by events which most people consider pleasure-producing and uplifting, you can usually be sure that this individual is suffering from Adrenal Syndrome.

Summary

No two Adrenal Syndrome patients have like conditions or react similarly to treatment because of differences in their heredity and stress. The disorder, it has been noted, most often passes from mother to daughter. A more severe appearance of the condition, called Chronic Adrenal Syndrome, may be recognized by a vacuity or glassiness of a patient's eyes and by extremely low blood pressure readings when the patient stands. Patients with Chronic Adrenal Syndrome, as a rule, become agitated if they have to wait, may go to great lengths emotionally in order to "awaken" adrenal function, and are unable to forget negative incidents. For Adrenal Syndrome patients relationships with others are often debilitiating. Crowds have a negative effect. Persons with Chronic Adrenal Syndrome don't react positively to surprises; they find that some friends weaken them, others strengthen them.

CHAPTER III

Clinical Treatment

In the treatment of Adrenal Syndrome, one of the first and most important factors is to assure the patient that he has a specific condition, that its cause is known, and that its correction is readily available to those who desire such help.

With many patients, it is obvious from the first interview that their condition is serious and that they are going to require the most complete treatment, including stress-reduction procedures. I usually make it a policy to be frank with these patients and let them know early what they and I must do.

In Adrenal Syndrome, as in most other diseases to which the body is subject, the patient's success in regaining health depends as much on his attitude and cooperation as on the skill and treatment of his physician. As I will point out throughout the text, however, the nature of Adrenal Syndrome makes it difficult for many patients to cooperate with their physician. For this reason, I sometimes impose conditions for treatment. I remember one severe patient whom I had refused to treat unless she stayed with us for six months of therapy. Her family fussed and fumed, but finally agreed. She returned home at the end of six months an entirely new person and remains so to this day. Had I equivocated on this case and tried less extensive treatment, I would have failed, and she would have given up long before improvement ensued.

The secret of all successful Adrenal Syndrome therapy can be illustrated by the Classic Double-Pan Scale (Figure 1) in which the total stresses of the patient are in one pan and the total treatment in the other. If the stress pan is heavier than the treatment pan, the patient will worsen. If less, the patient will improve, and, if equal, the patient will remain as he is, neither getting worse nor getting better.

Figure 1 illustrates that the amount of treatment must outweigh the force of the stresses which encumber the patient if treatment is to succeed. Successful therapy can be accomplished in three ways:

- Increase therapy until it is stronger than stresses.
- Decrease stress to a point at which the therapy is greater.
- Use methods which both increase therapy and lower stress.

An understanding of this balance mechanism allows great freedom

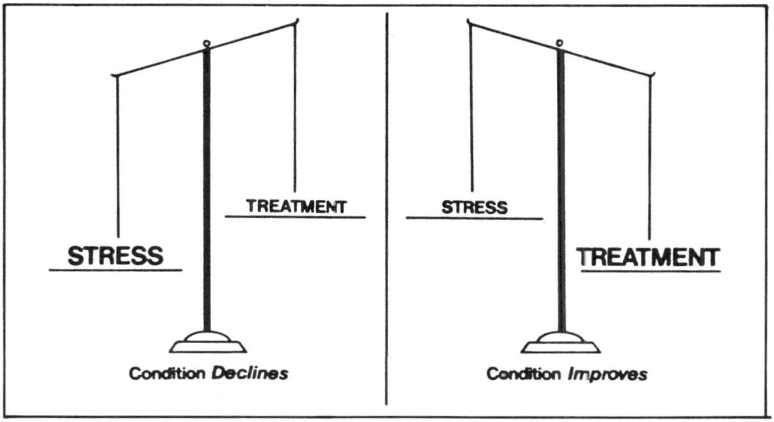

Figure 1. Classic Double-Pan Scale

and leeway in the type of therapy which is applied to an individual case. For instance, the low-income patient who cannot readily afford most of the forms of clinical therapy necessary for this condition can still be helped by counseling which will reduce the various stresses under which he lives. If the patient can reduce the amount of stress sufficiently, so it drops below the level of even minimal therapy, he will improve.

At the other extreme, patients often are in such an emotional state because of their condition that it is almost impossible for them to control their external and internal stresses. These patients come into the Clinic for complete inpatient care, so that they may receive careful personal management and an accelerated course of therapy to help support and regenerate the general adaptive mechanism.

It is also possible to treat two patients who are almost identical in their exposures to stress and their inherent glandular weaknesses successfully by what at first may appear to be entirely different therapy techniques. As we do this, we treat from different sides of the balance scale. In one case, because of certain extenuating circumstances, we might concentrate on stress reduction; in the other, clinical treatment might be the most expeditious approach. In fact, it is in knowing at which point to place the emphasis of treatment that the true skill of the physician is shown. The basic mechanisms of treating Adrenal Syndrome are simple and are fully outlined in this text. The difference between success and failure often depends on the experience and wisdom of the physician, on his knowledge of how to achieve that balance of clinical treatment and stress reduction that is best for the individual patient. Luckily, it is not absolutely essential for most patients to have exactly the correct proportions of these two factors to improve. The proper proportions do, however, give the most rapid and thorough improvement.

Specific Treatment Techniques

Specific clinical therapy can be divided into three components: internal, external, and counseling.

Internal includes specific nutritional and supportive agents which are supplied to the body to aid in its regeneration of the general adaptive mechanism.

External refers to treatment procedures and methods which are utilized to regenerate the general adaptive mechanism by means that do not require any substance to enter the body. Such treatments as Magnatherm,[1] Myoflex,[2] diathermy, hydrotherapy, remedial exercises, massage, and tissue sludge come under this classification.

The third division of clinical therapy is self-explanatory: counseling. Almost all clinical therapy would be worthless if the patients were not, first of all, properly counseled to have an understanding and appreciation of their condition, and then trained in the methods and techniques necessary to help them overcome the stresses which aggravate and prolong this problem.

Internal Therapies. *Diet.* The diet used for this condition is of great importance. I generally recommend a low-stress diet which provides, in as readily assimilable form as possible, all of the nutrient elements needed for satisfactory bodily function with special emphasis on those compounds which help to regenerate the general adaptive mechanism. The diet should be so arranged to include only the foods that are most easily digested, absorbed, and metabolized. It should exclude all foods that contain toxic substances which place added stress on the system and foods which require more energy to digest and assimilate than they return to the body in nutritive value. For the patient who does not have frank hypoglycemia, I usually use a combination of our Clinic's Basic Maintenance Diet and the Hypoglycemic Diet. (See Appendix I for diets.) The frequent meals, moderate protein, and increased intake of fruits and vegetables of the Hypoglycemic Diet seem to fit the needs of most Adrenal Syndrome

---

[1]Manufactured by International Medical Electronics, Ltd., 2805 Main Street, Kansas City, Missouri 64108.

[2]Manufactured by M.J. Edwards, 3515 Velva St., Shreveport, Louisiana 71109.

patients. In general, Adrenal Syndrome patients may have reasonable amounts of honey, dried fruits, rice, bananas, potatoes, and other similar foods which are usually excluded from the diet of true hypoglycemic patients.

The foods chosen should be as free of pesticides and additives as possible. Although organically grown foods are not an absolute prerequisite, we find that patients who are able to obtain and use organically grown foods or their home-grown counterparts recover more rapidly. Attempts should also be made to obtain chicken, fish, lean meat, and other proteins from as reliable a source as possible. Try to get them fresh and as free from chemical additives as possible since these substances are still being used in many of these products.

When the general adaptive mechanism begins to fail, one of the first body functions to be impeded is the digestive system. Therefore, most of these patients have digestive problems of a lesser or greater degree and it is all the more important that every mouthful of food these patients take be as nutritious and non-stress-producing as possible.

While the digestive mechanism is usually affected in most Adrenal Syndrome patients, it may be affected in different and sometimes diametrically opposite ways in individual patients. In some, the condition called anorexia, or poor appetitie, is present. These patients must be supplied with small but frequent amounts of highly nutritious foods. In others, the appetite becomes voracious, as if the body were attempting to make up in quantity what it lacks in quality. The new gastric analysis instrument, known as the "Heidelberg" pH monitoring instrument,[3] can be of great help in determining imbalances present in the individual patient's digestive system and in providing specific information as to what form of supplementation is needed to overcome his digestive dysfunctioning. Having this information is important, because in the healthy individual there is a balance of hydrochloric acid and the acidic-working enzymes of the stomach, the alkaline-working enzymes of the duodenum and small intestine, the fat-emulsifying elements from the gall bladder, and the bacterial breakdown of foods in the large intestine.

Normal digestion requires a proper synchronization of all of these factors. With the failure of the general adaptive mechanism, this synchronization frequently becomes disturbed. These patients are best helped by a rebalancing of this synchronization so that foods

[3]Manufactured by AEG-Telefunken, West Germany. Distributed by Electro-Medical Devices, Inc., Scientific Instruments Division, 6669 Peachtree Industrial Boulevard, Atlanta, Georgia 30092.

and supplements may be utilized to their best advantage. Many Adrenal Syndrome patients have great difficulty digesting and absorbing the specific supplements that are essential to improvement of their condition. For these patients, it is necessary to work on the digestive system before the internal portion of the clinical treatment can be instituted in a proper manner.

The pH monitoring instrument is extremely helpful in determining digestive system synchronization. With this diagnostic instrument, a special miniaturized radio transmitter and pH meter, no larger than a vitamin pill, is ingested and monitored by a special receiver-recorder as it passes through the digestive system. This little capsule sends out harmless radio signals to an instrument which graphs the changes in pH as it passes through the stages of digestion. The synchronous nature of the digestive system can be evaluated quite accurately by knowing the time intervals and the pH, that is, the degree of acid or alkaline, at any specific time. From this knowledge, the degree and nature of the imbalance can be calculated and necessary measures can be taken to correct it. This correction is accomplished by the use of various digestants, special food combinations, and therapy directed to the nerve centers in control of digestion.

Many patients with Adrenal Syndrome also have various food sensitivities. In these patients, even the best of regular diets can be injurious. Special testing must be done to ascertain the patient's needs. This is fully described in a later chapter.

Nutritional Supplements. Once the patient's dietary and digestive requirements are met, we are ready to look into his specific nutritional therapy. Proper supplemental therapy is probably the single most important clinical treatment component in the mild to moderate case. Without this therapy, it is rare for true and permanent improvement in the Adrenal Syndrome patient. It alone is sufficient to make dramatic improvement in many of the milder cases. In our Clinic, we usually use a supplement containing vitamin C, calcium pantothenate, vitamin B-6, and raw adrenal substance. This last compound, which is absolutely essential to proper adrenal regeneration, is made by dessicating a bovine adrenal gland at below body temperature so as not to destroy any of the delicate RNA and DNA factors necessary to help promote a rapid recovery from this condition. The product we most frequently use is called "Adrenucleo,"[4] a compound which contains all of the substances just mentioned plus

[4]Prepared by Enzyme Process Company, Inc., 19927 Bahama Street, Northridge, California 91324.

other compounds from natural sources used in its preparation. Occasionally, we use a product called "Drenamin,"[5] for patients who are sensitive to the fairly high doses of vitamin C contained in Adrenucleo. Drenamin mainly contains the dessicated adrenal gland substance without added amounts of specific vitamins. Recently we have been using a new, concentrated substance named "Mil-Adregen"[6] that seems to produce the same benefits of Adrenucleo and Drenamin, but at a lower dosage per day. The product itself is more expensive per tablet than both Adrenucleo and Drenamin, so there is no particular price saving, but for patients who find the high dosages of Drenamin and Adrenucleo necessary for proper recovery a chore to take the lower dosage item, Mil-Adregen, may be the remedy of choice.

Possibly due to some of the pioneering work performed on this condition at the Clymer Health Clinic, more nutritional supplement producers are introducing to the market compounds designed to regenerate the general adaptive mechanism. The only products for whose integrity I can personally vouch are the three mentioned above. This is not to say that other products may not be of help. I have not had sufficient experience with them to make a recommendation. It is not sufficient to merely capsule adrenal gland substance and purport to have a product to aid in the regeneration of the Adrenal Syndrome patient. Many vital factors in these substances are easily destroyed by improper extraction or manufacturing methods. At this time we have no way of analyzing whether these newer products contain the elements which will help these patients. Only through clinical experience can this information be gained. Because of this fact, please do not judge the effectiveness of the treatment recommended in this text unless you are using the *specific compounds* which I recommend. They are the only ones that I *know* will work.

Next to the adrenal gland substance supplement, I find the elements of the vitamin B-complex family most vital. The compound which has proven the most effective for me is "B-Plus,"[7] which is derived from a combination of natural sources: yeast, liver, and rice-bran concentrates. This product contains many of the coenzymes not present in purified formulations, which, in my experience, are

[5]Prepared by Standard Process Laboratories, Inc., Division of Vitamin Products, Co., Milwaukee, Wisconsin 53207.

[6]Prepared by Miller Pharmaceutical Group, Inc., 245 West Roosevelt, (P.O. Box 279), West Chicago, Illinois 60185.

[7]Prepared by Enzyme Process Company, Inc., 19927 Bahama Street, Northridge, California 91324.

essential to proper adrenal regeneration. B-Plus also contains other glandular extracts which help provide a multiple glandular support of the general adaptive mechanism. Thus, we are providing the plural-glandular technique so much favored by Dr. Henry Harrower in his work, *Practical Organic Therapy, The Internal Secretions in General Practice* (1). I have not found an effective substitute for B-Plus and, therefore, cannot recommend any other product as having the same beneficial effect for the Adrenal Syndrome patient.

These two compounds are the minimum internal supplemental therapy that I recommend for the Adrenal Syndrome patient. This is often sufficient for mild cases, but patients who have more severe symptoms require additional supplementation. The substance usually given next is vitamin B-15. The chemical name of this compound is calcium pangamate or pangamic acid. Here, again, we have found that many of the so-called B-15 or calcium pangamate products on the market do not bring the proper benefit to the patient. At the time of publication of this book, the product I have found most successful is "Gluconic 15."[8] Vitamin B-15 acts as a catalyst in the system; that is, it is a compound which assists in carrying out a chemical reaction while it is not a part of the reaction. Although there is no way of knowing all the specific reactions it promotes, experience has proven that in patients on B-15 regeneration takes place faster than in those without it.

Adrenal Syndrome often occurs in those of low income. Unless the condition is quite severe, we try to restrict low-income patients to the above internal therapy. If we subject a patient to costs he is not readily able to pay, we create in him a stress that tends to worsen his condition. Thus, it is easy to aggravate the very condition we are trying to correct. This factor is not always taken into account by many clinics who attempt to treat this condition, and yet it has an undeniable effect on the patient's state of improvement.

If a patient is able to afford it, we recommend a specific analysis of his supplemental needs by the use of a screening test, which we developed at the Clymer Health Clinic, called the "General Nutritional Profile" (also termed "General Metabolic Profile"). In this procedure, special examinations of the blood, urine, hair, and diet are made, which provide us with a detailed report of the patient's individual body's deficiencies and imbalances. Following the completion of this testing procedure, it is a simple matter to suggest the specific diet and/or nutritional substances need to aid in

---

[8]Produced by DaVinci Laboratories, 1 Executive Drive, Burlington, Vermont 05401.

rebalancing the body's chemistries. In moderate to severe Adrenal Syndrome cases such procedures are absolutely essential.[9]

To understand the need for such balancing of the body, we must, once again, return to the analogy shown in Figure 1. Any reduction of stress helps the Adrenal Syndrome patient recover more rapidly. By analyzing his body's chemistry and creating optimal nutritional balance within his system, one form of stress is reduced—which can be extremely important in certain instances and useful in all.

Adrenal Cortical Extract. Once the dietary and supplemental requirements of the patient are met, one rather controversial form of internal therapy remains. That is, the use of adrenal cortical extract (ACE) injections. Other injectable agents have proven useful in the treatment of Adrenal Syndrome, and they will be discussed here also. To understand the value as well as the possible misuse of adrenal cortical extract, we must review the functioning of the adrenal glands in these patients.

In normal functioning, the adrenal glands work similarly to that of a thermostatically controlled furnace. When the heat in the home drops below a certain level, the furnace starts and continues until the temperature rises to a certain predetermined level, at which point the furnace shuts itself off and remains off until the temperature again reaches the thermostatically controlled lower-level setting at which the furnace again turns on. In the properly functioning furnace, this procedure is carried on ad infinitum as weather and outside temperature require. The adrenal glands, as well as most other endocrine glands of the body, are controlled by a similar mechanism. The body requires for its general functioning a certain level of cortical hormones. Normal adrenal glands release these hormonal substances into the bloodstream when the level in the blood reaches a point below which the body can function optimally. The adrenal glands continue to secrete these substances until a certain preset level is reached at which point, like the furnace, it shuts off, not to resume secretion until the hormones in the bloodstream reach the previously mentioned low point again. Then, as the furnace, they begin to secrete anew and continue to repeat this process as need arises.

There are two basic ways in which the ACE may be used for Adrenal Syndrome patients. The first is as a massive replacement therapy to augment regular adrenal functioning. The second

[9]This one point of therapy is so vital to the recovery from Adrenal Syndrome that the entire next chapter is devoted to it.

technique is to use it to allow rest periods for the adrenal glands so that they may regenerate. In the first instance, large amounts of ACE—from 10cc to 20cc—are injected into the venous system once or twice a week. Many doctors have in the past used this procedure for treating hypoglycemia with some success. (My own feeling is that they were actually treating the low adrenal functioning which many feel is the cause of hypoglycemia.)

Large Dosages of ACE. The injection of large amounts of adrenal cortical extract into the venous system can be therapeutically dramatic and may be essential in certain severe, acute states of Adrenal Syndrome. But for the average chronic patient under long-term care it has certain drawbacks, which I feel negate its usefulness. I do not feel that it is physiologically sound therapy for chronic cases. As mentioned earlier, all endocrine glands are stimulated by a demand mechanism. That is, they are stimulated to secrete when the blood levels of their hormones reach a certain low point and to shut off when these levels reach another somewhat higher point. If massive amounts of a gland's secretions are given to the body on a regular basis, the gland will be inhibited to such an extent that it will stop producing adequate amounts of its own secretions. This is basic human physiology. If large amounts of ACE are continually pumped into a patient's bloodstream, he will feel better, it is true, and the adrenal glands will be shut off and allowed to rest. This in itself is beneficial, but, if injection of these amounts is continued, the gland no longer has a need to produce its own secretions. The demand mechanism will not trigger, because of the high levels of ACE in the bloodstream. If this high dosage of ACE is continued for an extended period of time, the adrenal gland possibly could reach a state at which it could not regenerate. While this may not occur in every case, and may not occur as often as we fear, we are meddling with a delicate balance.

Another problem with the intravenous injection of ACE is that it makes the patient too dependent on the doctor. In our work, we attempt to make patients as independent as possible. Only by building up their confidence in themselves and their own abilities as individuals can we truly reduce and keep minimal the various stresses which they must confront as functioning human beings. The more they depend on other individuals, even their doctor, the more difficult it is to reach this state.

Another important factor is the high cost of adrenal cortical extract; it is not an inexpensive remedy and, used in such large amounts, can be an inordinate financial drain on the patient.

I personally recommend this procedure only for a patient who is overwhelmed by unremitting stress from which he cannot extricate himself due to factors not under his own personal control and for whom all other methods of therapy have not been adequate to tip the scales in his favor. In twenty-five years of treating these cases, I luckily have found few patients who fell into this extreme category. Even in these few severe instances, the patients were kept on the massive dosage for only a short time. As soon as possible the patient was placed on the lower dosage ACE and/or oral therapy.

Patients with severe symptoms might be treated with cortisone by an orthodox practitioner; while I am not enamored with the use of large dosages of ACE, it is far less toxic than the cortisone compounds.

There is one other time at which large doses of ACE have been found helpful—in the differential diagnosis of Adrenal Syndrome from those conditions which may mimic it. If the true Adrenal Syndrome patient is given an injection of 10cc to 20cc of 2-X ACE, he should notice considerable improvement in his entire being within a few minutes to hours. This improvement should last a day or two, at least, and then gradually subside. Should the patient notice no improvement from this amount of ACE, the adrenal component of his problem is probably not the major cause of his symptoms, and the health professional should look to food allergies, defects in brain nutrition, hypoglycemia, hypothyroidism, or other related difficulties.

LOW DOSE USAGE OF ACE. In our Clinic, we have perfected a low-dosage use of adrenal cortical extract which seems to overcome the difficulties encountered with the large-dosage intravenous method and which is capable of providing practically all of the therapeutic value of the large dose, especially for the chronic case. As used in our Clinic, the purpose of the adrenal cortical extract is *not* to supplant the secretions of the person's own glands. It is used mainly as a method of permitting the adrenal glands to rest. I stress this point because many patients expect to feel better as soon as they start to receive the injections, only to discover that they are sometimes more exhausted and less capable of pushing themselves than they were before this treatment started. This is the desired result and is easily explained if we examine the physiology of the matter. By these injections, we attempt to raise the level of the adrenal cortical hormones in the blood to the point at which the adrenal glands shut off for a period of rest. This is essential for adrenal recovery because *only* during periods when the adrenal glands are at rest are they capable of regeneration. There is no chance of improvement for the patient who cannot obtain these important periods of adrenal rest.

At times, the exhaustion following the first ACE shots persists and is explainable by the fact that once a gland that has been running without rest shuts off, it is often difficult for it to start up again. It is like an individual who has gone several days without sleep; once he goes to sleep, he may sleep for an inordinately long time and be difficult to arouse. The adrenal glands so need this rest that often the levels of the hormone in the blood drop below the normal turn-on point before this resting gland reactivates itself. During this period in which the blood levels of the cortical hormones are low, the patient feels much more tired and exhausted than usual. It can be a good exhaustion, however. By that I mean, an exhaustion without the anxiety which is produced by the constantly running weakened adrenal glands. Unfortunately, all too many Adrenal Syndrome patients expect a rapid and uneventful recovery and consider good only that which produces in them what they call a normal feeling; that is, the feeling which is present with full functioning adrenal hormones in the blood. This feeling can and will come to every adrenal patient who is treated properly, but it does not usually come by proper therapeutic use of adrenal cortical extract alone.

Not all patients with this state of increased exhaustion respond to ACE. In fact, the degree of depth of Adrenal Syndrome is indicated by the patient's reaction to small amounts of ACE. If the patient feels a lift from an injection, I consider the case mild and easy to cure because the level of hormone is near normal, and the addition of a small amount of ACE raised his hormonal level to a degree sufficient to create a symptomatic improvement.

Patients who notice no real effect from ACE injections—and these are the great majority—I consider to be moderately severe. In these patients, the adrenal hormone is low enough so that the addition of a small amount of ACE in the body does not make sufficient change to produce an immediate alleviation of the symptoms. On the other hand, the adrenal gland is not so weakened that it cannot respond once the level of body hormones reaches the turn-on point.

When a patient experiences increased exhaustion after receiving ACE, we consider his case to be more serious because his adrenals are not capable of resuming activity when the hormone levels are low.

The ACE most often is given in dosages ranging from 1cc to 4cc, using the 2-X variety. Dosage is repeated from as often as daily to as infrequently as once a month, depending on the severity and state of recovery of the patient.

Not all Adrenal Syndrome patients require ACE and our general clinical policy is to treat the patient by the most natural, least harmful, and most inexpensive approach possible. Over the years, we, at the Clinic, have become known for our treatment of this condition, and we do attract more of the serious, chronic-type patients and, in these instances, ACE is frequently a vital factor in their recovery.

Certain other substances have been found to be beneficial when given in conjunction with ACE. These include such nutritional compounds as "Calphosan." which is a calcium compound,[10] vitamin B-12, vitamin B-6, vitamin B-1, and raw crude liver.

External Clinical Treatment. The most misunderstood and unappreciated part of the treatment of Adrenal Syndrome is the external clinical treatment. It is not difficult to explain to a patient suffering from this complaint how various stress-reducing procedures are going to help him. Most of us are accustomed to taking pills and injections, and we have little difficulty in understanding how this type of therapy is going to help. But many find it difficult to understand how a machine can help regenerate their adrenal glands. Nevertheless, the external treatment is usually a must for speedy recovery.

Machines. The two most useful machines (I like to call them "regenerative therapy instruments," but my patients insist on calling them "machines") which we use are the Magnatherm and the Myoflex. They have a similar purpose, although they work on entirely different principles. The Magnatherm produces a pulsating electromagnetic energy, while the Myoflex effects a complex multiple sine-wave current which is designed to mimic the energy produced by the human nerve cell.

Before I go into detail about these two instruments, I wish to mention other methods of external treatment. If muscle tension and spasm have been produced from long-encountered bodily stress, the standard diathermy and/or sine-wave machines are often helpful in reducing this problem. When muscle tension is accompanied by nervous irritation, such external therapies as the whirlpool bath, sauna, wet-sheet pack, and various forms of massage are extremely helpful. All these are effective, predicated on an understanding of the basic premise stated at the beginning of this chapter. Any form of treatment which produces a reduction of stress in the body, mind, or soul relieves the general adaptive system, and, therefore, helps Adrenal Syndrome.

---

[10]Produced by Carlton Corporation, 83 North Summit Street, Tenafly, New Jersey 07670.

While the Magnatherm and the Myoflex may seem at first to be similar to the other therapies I have just discussed, the basic mechanism of their functioning is different. The purpose of the Magnatherm and Myoflex treatments is not to reduce stress on the body; it is actually to encourage the regeneration of the bodily organs. These instruments, in my experience, have the capability of helping to regenerate organs and tissues that are not, under the present state of the body, able to regenerate themselves. In the case of Adrenal Syndrome, we treat the liver, spleen, adrenals, and both kidneys. This method encompasses a great deal of the reticuloendothelial system and helps to mobilize the general adaptive system. Can I prove that they work? I only know that for the past twenty-five years I have been constantly experimenting and refining the treatment of this condition. Many therapies have been tried; many therapies have been discarded. The ones that I use now have, at least, stood the test of time.

Some patients with severe allergic sensitivities produced by Adrenal Syndrome are able to take almost no internal medication without severe reaction. The only clinical therapy possible is the "machines." These trustworthy servants have never yet let me down. Usually after a short time the patient improves sufficiently to be able to begin internal treatment and go on to ultimate recovery. From time to time a patient does not make the progress that I expect, and I am concerned because, with the therapy and counseling he receives, he should be better. Almost invariably, upon querying him about the machine treatment, I have found that due to lack of time on his part, or more generally due to a misunderstanding of the value of these treatments, he has not been taking the recommended Myoflex and Magnatherm treatments. Once these treatments again become a regular part of his therapy, his progress returns to a normal rate. The Magnatherm and Myoflex both work by directing the healing forces of the body to specific areas of need. They also have an effect on the electronic nature of the cell and, through this influence, stimulate cellular regeneration. Such cell-level regeneration is difficult to prove, however, so we let the results speak for themselves.

Manual Therapies. In *It's Only Natural* I wrote about the use of certain physical therapy methods in Adrenal Syndrome (2). I find the comments perfectly valid today, and, therefore, repeat them without change.

> It's been my observation that most hypoadrenal cases also have nerve-muscle-bone displacements and tensions in the area of the shoulder blade and along the upper thoracic and lower neck areas. These we treat with mild ultrasound therapy and with finger

pressure, working the sensitive areas to gradually eliminate the nerve-muscle spasms and in turn any bony displacements. In some of the more sensitive patients, this work must be handled with great delicacy; but as improvement occurs the pressure may be increased. In fact, we find that as the adrenal condition of our patient improves, he becomes less and less sensitive to this treatment and he finds it increasingly more pleasant.

The explanation for the relief from soreness in the upper back and neck that patients receive from this simple maneuver is simple. When the glandular system is low, lactic acid and other acid metabolites tend to accumulate in the muscle areas of the shoulder and upper back. The ultrasound therapy and finger pressure break up the acid deposits so they are free to return to the circulating blood to be eliminated from the body by the usual routes of elimination. While this is an apparently simple component of our therapy, many patients find it a necessary one. I particularly recall two patients, a mother and her daughter, whom I had been treating for some time. The treatment had been long and slow due to a constant, unremitting stress factor at home which simply was not capable of change or improvement. At one time in their treatment, however, I noticed—by the look in their eyes—that they both seemed to be going down hill. At that time, I sat down with them and went over every component of their treatment. They were taking all of the forms of internal therapies; they were taking the machine therapies; and they were coming twice a week which was even more than I had asked. The only thing that they were not doing was getting the massage and manipulative therapy because they thought it would prolong their visits. I persuaded them to start this part of the therapy once again to see if it would aid in their improvement. With the first treatment they felt better. By the end of two weeks they were nearly back to their old selves. Since the stress at home had not changed, I continued to see them as patients. But they remained in a much improved condition and were sure each time to get their full manipulative and massage therapies.

Spinal manipulation, while different from the tissue sludge technique described above, has always proven to be a useful and important part of the clinical treatment of this syndrome. It has several factors going for it. It can be a great reducer of both physical and emotional stress. Both emotional and mental stress produces tension in the body's physical structures. This tension manifests itself most commonly around the neck, shoulders, and back areas. All of these areas are intimately associated with the spine and its adjacent structures. By freeing the physical manifestation of the tension, there is a reduction in the tendency for the nervous stress to reproduce itself continuously. If we become upset or tense through some nervous stress or tension, our physical structure may go into spasm, which produces tension on the nerves and other allied soft tissues. Such physical tension can reduce a patient's basic feeling of well-being. By lowering his feeling of well-being, he becomes more susceptible to nervous and emotional stress, which, in turn, produces more physical stress, which, in turn, further reduces his well-being—producing a vicious circle which must be broken somewhere along its course to enable him to feel well again.

One of the simplest and most productive methods of restoring the patient's feeling of well-being is to break up the physical tensions that occur in the body. This is one of the most important values of all forms of manipulative therapies—massage, deep-muscle treatments, and even various exercise programs. The now-popular jogging and running procedures also have a somewhat similar effect, although they are not as specific as the use of spinal manipulation and deep massage.

Medical authorities to the contrary, there are such things as vertebral subluxations, that is, a spinal segment out of alignment. This misalignment can be a primary cause of physical stresses and the only way that these can be reduced is by spinal manipulation. Many patients with Adrenal Syndrome cannot obtain full recovery until certain spinal misalignments are corrected by a series of spinal manipulations.

Various forms of massage, hydrotherapy, and other therapies in use at the Clinic fall into the category of stress-reducing external techniques. They all have their place. Their effectiveness in each case varies with the nature of the individual. Sometimes half an hour with our massage therapist does more good than almost any other form of treatment. Other patients do not want to be touched by anyone, and the same massage therapy which was so efficacious for one would create severe tension in another. There is no specific therapy for the Adrenal Syndrome patient. There are basic guidelines, however, which must be followed: Reduce stress as much as possible, then support and regenerate the general adaptive mechanism. The methods by which these two goals are accomplished in any individual case must always be left to the discernment and discrimination of the doctor handling that patient. To paraphrase the Bible: "One patient's cure is another patient's stress."

Perhaps it is this inability to prescribe a specific useful treatment for each patient with this condition that has made the disease so difficult to recognize and accept by most practitioners. It may be why they prefer not to accept such cases. Not long ago a patient from Pittsburgh, Pennsylvania, who had a severe case of adrenal exhaustion, asked me to find a doctor nearer his home. I gave him names of several doctors whom I knew should be able to treat his disease, but in each instance, as soon as the physician discovered the patient had adrenal symptoms, he refused to accept him as a patient.

Therapeutic Counseling. "He that can't be counseled, can't be helped."—BENJAMIN FRANKLIN.

The most vital treatment for the chronic adrenal case is patient counseling. Before we can fully appreciate the importance and value of counseling for Adrenal Syndrome patients, we should visualize what has usually happened to these patients before they come under this therapy. Strange and enigmatic symptoms began and gradually intensified in these persons. They sought help from this doctor and that doctor, from this psychologist and that psychologist, trying to find an answer to problems. Usually, each professional gave them a different answer. In each instance, a different therapy was tried, with little or no improvement. Many sufferers were assured during these periods that they had a mental difficulty. Most tried so many different therapies without real success that by the time they come to us they are ready to accept a diagnosis of mental illness and are afraid to expect improvement for fear of once again having their hopes dashed. Their friends and relatives are eager to give them advice, none of which seems to help—in fact, all of which seems to depress them further. They are in truth the emotional dregs of society. Their self-confidence and emotional stability, on a scale of one to ten, usually are at a minus six. If ever patients were in need of counseling and some kind words, these are the ones.

Once the diagnosis is finalized, counseling should begin. Several specific objectives are to be obtained by counseling, the first and foremost of which is to explain his condition to the patient. Before he can be helped, the patient must accept the diagnosis and understand the character of Adrenal Syndrome. It is imperative that he realize that it is a physical condition which, even though it may have been with him for many years, is treatable and correctable. Strange to say, as good as this news is, it is difficult for most people to accept. They usually are locked into one of two diametrically opposite patterns of thought. In one group are persons who are not willing to accept that they have this type of condition, which requires a lengthy and extensive treatment, but vainly hope that it is merely a vitamin or mineral deficiency which, once detected and corrected, will let them become their old selves in a few days. At the other end are those who are positive that the condition is really a mental disease or of such a nature that it is untreatable, so there is no real hope for them. The truth, of course, lies somewhere between. It is the obligation and duty of the doctor to constantly reiterate this fact until the patient truly understands and accepts the nature of the condition.

In the first instance, the patients constantly say to themselves, "There's nothing really that much wrong with me. I've just got some little problem that is making me tired. If I just get enough rest, I'll come out of it; if I can just find that right vitamin or that misssing mineral; or if some doctor would give me the right adjustment, then I'll be better." They expect a cure without any real effort on their parts. Patients of the first group are not willing to accept the condition mainly because such acceptance requires them to acknowledge a degree of problem they wish to deny. Such acceptance requires a change in their life habits and a certain amount of dedication to overcome the difficulty. It is hard for many to accept that they have certain hereditary weaknesses in their glandular systems, but, until they do, there can be no real help for them—here or elsewhere. Many times patients, whom I had diagnosed as having Adrenal Syndrome, left, unconvinced, to seek other opinions only to return months or years later in far worse condition. They were at last willing to accept my diagnosis, having failed to find help elsewhere. Unfortunately, they then were much more difficult to treat because the condition had progressed considerably.

Patients in the second category usually readily accept the fact that they have the condition. But their attitude often is, "Oh, I probably have it all right, but I know I'll never get over it." The situation is right back where it started because the whole purpose of getting patient acceptance is to obtain patient cooperation for treatment, and they have given up before they started. Without patient cooperation, any treatment is long and protracted because, for adequate patient response, the patient must realize what he has, accept what he has, acknowledge that the treatment can overcome the condition, and work with the doctor toward this end. It is the counselor's job to convince these patients that they can be helped.

Once patient acceptance has been achieved, special counseling is begun to reduce emotional and psychological stresses that are present in the patient. This procedure can be one of the most time-consuming, grueling, and yet rewarding procedures involved in the treatment of Adrenal Syndrome.

Types of Stress. There are three basic types of stress which the patient can manifest. The first is physical stress; the second, mental stress; and the third, emotional stress. The least damaging is physical stress; next comes mental stress, and the most harmful and far-reaching is emotional stress. In our counseling sessions we deal with emotional stress.

Many patients ask how to differentiate between mental stress and emotional stress. Mental stress is stress produced from reading, doing income taxes, or balancing a bank book—stress caused by using the mind as a functioning element. Emotional stress includes, of course, those things which affect the emotions, such as fear, jealousy, anger, revenge, resentment, or worry. Something which triggers the emotions is different from that which is merely the use of the brain for mental work. Physical stress is, of course, obviously simply the functioning of the muscular system of the body.

While on the subject of these three types of stresses, I might mention that in therapy, if a patient has a choice of exchanging one stress for the other, he should attempt to exchange them in the reverse order from which they have been listed here. In other words, if it is possible to exchange a mental stress for an emotional stress, he should go ahead and do it; he will gain from it. If he can exchange a physical stress for an emotional stress, it is a good exchange. An example of such an exchange would be a patient who loves to go dancing but who overextends herself and exhausts her adrenal glands. However, she may be looking forward to a special dance so much that if she did not go, an emotional stress would be created that would probably outweigh the physical stress that she might experience by going. In this instance, it is wiser for her to go to the dance and exchange a physical stress for an emotional one.

This same circumstance is often true regarding patients and their employment. The nature of physical and mental stresses involved in their work tends to slow their recovery from Adrenal Syndrome. However, their sense of family responsibilities and the nature of their individual character may be such that, were they prevented from working, the emotional stresses of not being productive and being financially depressed may be far greater than the physical and the mental damage done by working. In these and similar instances, it is better to substitute one of the less damaging stresses for those more damaging.

Likewise with exercise. In fact, one of the most common questions I am asked by Adrenal Syndrome patients is: "How much exercise should I take?" For the Adrenal Syndrome patient, exercise must be considered as a physical stress and treated accordingly. This does not mean it should not be attempted—after all, physical stress is the least of the stesses—only that the patient must take certain precautions in its use. The master rule is: *As long as you feel no weakness or exhaustion the day after exercise, you are all right and have not overdone. One the other hand, if you do feel exhaustion after exercise, you have done too much.* The patient who has overdone must learn to reduce future exercise programs until he no longer experiences the exhaustion. In this manner, each Adrenal Syndrome patient can find the optimal amount of exercise which is best for him. As the patient improves, neuroglandular tone is gained, and the amount of exercise performed can be gradually increased. The amount of increase may once again be ascertained by the procedure outlined above.

The Power of the Truth. In counseling for stress reduction, each patient is an individual problem, although some basic rules apply. It is important to build true rapport between the clinician and the patient. To this end, nothing is so powerful as the truth. I make it an unbreakable rule never to lie even in the slightest detail to an Adrenal Syndrome patient. This penchant for truth must be carried to the point where the clinician must want to help this patient; the clinician has to like this patient. If he cannot, it is probably wisest to refer the patient to another doctor. To become a patient's healer, a clinician must become his friend. Almost no one else understands these patients. They are in a small lonely boat floating in a sea of disbelief. The healer must constantly let them know that he understands their situation and that not only is he willing to help them, but that he has the skill, knowledge, and ability to do so. They require constant reassurance of the fact that they are going to get well and, to give them this reassurance, the clinician must have the knowledge to get them well. Unless he can say it from the heart, it will not be effective. People who are ill, and particularly individuals with Adrenal Syndrome, are quick to pick up any sign of indifference on the part of their practitioners.

Once a professional has earned their confidence, he can begin to dissect and treat their various stresses one by one. Sometimes, due to certain circumstances, major stresses cannot be approached at the beginning. The stresses may be too fearful for the patient to face or be of such a nature that the patient cannot yet accept their true character. Do not become discouraged if response is slow. Start with small treatable stresses. As the little stresses are worked out, and the patient gains more confidence in the healer, and as the rest of the therapeutic regime strengthens the patient's adaptive mechanisms, the time will come when together the clinician and the patient can confront larger stresses.

I always think of my patients as beautiful jewels covered with a pile of garbage. Each stress I help to remove is more garbage pulled off the pile. Eventually, I know, I will get to the jewel. Some pieces of garbage are small and some are large, but they all have to come off. Each one, no matter how small, moves me closer to the beauty of the jewel which I know is there.

Another general rule I use in this type of counseling is to always go forward, never back. I do not know how many times in my professional life I have quoted the biblical statement, "Let the dead bury the dead." That which has happened is done and gone; you cannot change it. The only thing that you can do is to go forward by obeying further another biblical command, "Follow thou me." Many Chronic Adrenal Syndrome patients have never really known a normal existence. They must build a new life, but to do this work, they must always proceed forward.

Group Therapy. In many instances, Adrenal Syndrome patients seem to benefit from association with other similar patients. In many of our programs, we utilize a form of group therapy to help them in their recovery. Unfortunately, much care must be taken with this therapy. One must understand the various mechanisms involved, and each patient must evaluate the effect upon his own being before he enters into any situation from which he cannot rapidly extricate himself.

One of the most common problems of the Adrenal Syndrome patient is the loneliness he feels. It seems to him that all of his friends are normal and that he alone has this problem which no one whom he knows seems to understand or appreciate. Also, not having anyone with whom to compare notes, the patient cannot gauge the extent of his recovery or see evidence of anyone's recovering. The Adrenal Syndrome patient is like a person at the bottom of a deep well. All he sees above him is a small, round shaft of light. His physician can tell him that there is a whole world of flowers, sunshine, and beauty out there once he climbs to the top of the well, but it is hard for him to believe while he is still at the bottom of the well. To be introduced to someone who has successfully climbed out of the well and emerged into the sunshine would be a great boost to this struggling patient.

If at the same time the patient can find a companion who has recovered or is on the way to recovery from Adrenal Syndrome, so much the better. In this way the patient has someone who can understand his feelings and who can reassure him by example. An important part of the cure is often accomplished by the camaraderie which can be established among Adrenal Syndrome patients. The main caution in this therapy is to prevent a weak patient from attaching himself to a stronger patient, almost like a leech, then expecting the stronger patient to help him through every little difficulty in his own life. Such practice can place an unfair stress on the stronger patient and lead to retrogression in his condition. The wise clinician constantly watches that one patient does not grow stronger by leeching strength from another.

The physician also watches for conflicting personalities among the patients. Sometimes two patients have the same condition and, therefore, have a certain empathy for one another. Yet by nature their personalities may be so different that one actually preys upon the other. In this situation it would be unwise to suggest that they attempt to help one another. When one directs an inpatient care facility, as I do at the Clymer Health Clinic, one must keep an eternal vigil for destructive interworkings between patients.

The nature of many Adrenal Syndrome patients makes them sacrificing, helpful individuals. It is usually this sacrificing nature which produces many of the stresses which brought about the condition in the first place. Such a patient must be taught to respect his own needs and health care first, for if he will not do this, he will not have the strength and energy necessary to help other people. In these circumstances, little is gained by sacrificing one's own strength in an attempt to aid another person. It is the responsibility of every Adrenal Syndrome patient to build his own individual strength, not to sap that of others. Unless the patient can do this, he will not have a permanent recovery or cure.

Clinical Integration. The steps outlined above constitute the general clinical therapeutic program for Adrenal Syndrome patients. One aspect of the program however, has not been discussed. All parts must be integrated into a whole and, particularly in severe cases, given to the patient under a situation of complete clinical control. We do that by bringing these patients into our Clinic for shorter or longer periods of composite treatment. Most patients with severe cases stay at our inpatient facility for a week or two to set up the necessary procedures and to begin preliminary counseling. If the case is not too severe, patients may then continue the proper therapy on an outpatient basis. The more severe cases may need to stay with us for extended periods, often one to three months. During this time, we are able to provide total commitment care, in which we control the entertainment they see, the food they eat, the air they breathe, and the water they drink. In severe Chronic Adrenal Syndrome patients, only this total patient care is adequate to give improvement. Such patient care must not only be

total, but individual. For example, Adrenal Syndrome patients who produce stress just waiting for their treatments are allowed to remain in their rooms until their treatments are ready so that they may rest as much as possible. Such measures, I am sure, seem extreme. They are necessary, however, for some severe adrenal cases. With diligence and persistence even these patients once again may return to normal functioning.
(See Appendix II for a word about the Clymer Health Clinic.)

One Step at a Time. As mentioned in his *Autobiography,* there was a time when Benjamin Franklin decided to overcome all his bad habits (3). However, try as he would, he found it almost impossible to be good all of the time. He discovered that he could not concentrate on more than one bad habit at a time. Using these principles, he evolved a technique in which he wrote down all his bad habits and each week concentrated his whole being on one habit and attempted to eliminate it. His presumption was that, having worked hard on the habit for seven days, a certain amount of habitual remembrance would be produced in his system so that as he tackled a new habit, some of the good gained in fighting the old habit would remain. Franklin continued this procedure for the rest of his life and, as he stated, he was able to control all of his habits except that of pride. He assumed that even if he was finally able to overcome pride, he would be too proud of his accomplishment to qualify for a real elimination.

In working with the stresses of the Adrenal Syndrome patient, a similar technique is most effective. By taking one stress at a time, a patient can frequently conquer where only failure met him previously.

I am reminded of a recent patient who had a bad smoking habit, drank ten cups of coffee a day, and had been on Valium® for many years. Any one of these habits would have been sufficient to prevent the progress of her condition, but all three made improvement difficult indeed. All attempts by former physicians had failed. By following Franklin's method, we were able to work her off coffee first, then cigarettes, and at last Valium®. Handling her in this manner, we were able to eliminate these noxious habits and finally treat and cure the Adrenal Syndrome itself.

Many patients who come to us have suffered from Adrenal Syndrome for many years. When they discover the length of time necessary for recovery, they often become discouraged. If they are willing to take their stresses one by one and work to correct them, they will see improvement in the entire being within a relatively short time. As they start to see these changes, they will develop enthusiasm for becoming an individual whose potential they had only previously imagined. According to a Chinese proverb, "A journey of a thousand miles starts with a single step." So it is with all of our stresses. We must take them one by one; work on one and improve it before we go on to the next. No one can stop all of the stresses in his life at once. We are, after all, only human beings, but, by being human, we have free will and indomitable courage that will hold us in good stead as we work toward overcoming the various conditions which assault our bodies, minds, and souls.

Summary

The first step in the clinical treatment of Adrenal Syndrome is to assure the patient that he has a specific condition which can be treated. In dealing with Adrenal Syndrome, another important factor is to reduce stress—emotional, mental, and physical—through integrated use of internal and external therapies and therapeutic counseling. In internal treatment, attention is given to diet and to nutritional supplements, both devised specifically for each individual patient. External treatment includes manual therapy and use of instruments. Therapeutic counseling, like the other treatment techniques, is individually oriented and is one of the most important aspects of the treatment regime. Throughout the patient's entire program of regaining health and stability he must be accepting of his condition and make an effort to progress one step at a time.

CHAPTER IV

Nutritional Imbalances and Deficiencies

The concept of nutritional imbalances and deficiencies often is disputed in the treatment of Adrenal Syndrome, as it is in the treatment and prevention of all conditions in the whole kaleidoscope of modern medicine. On one hand, there are physicians who contend that nutritional imbalances and deficiencies are the cause of nearly every disease known to mankind. On the other hand, there is that phalanx of medical orthodoxy which holds that, except for a few rare diseases, usually present only in other countries, such nutritional imbalances or deficiencies play little part in modern medicine. This disparity is somewhat similar to the controversy on hypoglycemia in that the truth lies undoubtedly somewhere between the two extremes. One wonders who in the long run does the greatest disservice to the honest promulgation of nutritional information, those who oversell this component of medicine or those who blatantly disregard it.

Importance of Therapeutic Balance

The correction of deficiencies and the establishment of a proper nutritional balance in the blood and tissues of Adrenal Syndrome patients is absolutely essential to their recovery. Unless this is accomplished, all other treatment work can be much prolonged and, in certain instances, thwarted entirely. However, proper ingestion and absorption of the nutritional elements necessary to build the general adaptive mechanism are not in themselves sufficient to correct this syndrome.

The analogy I use to illustrate this conclusion is that of building a house. Proper nutritional needs of a patient are analogous to the materials necessary for proper house construction. Lumber, cement blocks, mortar, electrical wiring, plumbing supplies, and roofing material are equivalent to the food we eat.

In the body, as in the house, several considerations enter into the selection of the building material. We must know what kind of a house we are building. Is it a Spanish ranch house, a stone Victorian mansion, or perhaps a Colonial saltbox? Obviously, the type of materials we select depends on the nature of the house. Each person's body is as different as these houses. Just as we would not order great amounts of brick and stone to build a Colonial saltbox, so we must be careful which specific nutrients we recommend for the Adrenal Syndrome patient.

A builder, in choosing the materials for his house, orders the finest he can afford, those which are going to build a solid, enduring structure. To do less would be false economy indeed, for his house would no sooner be built than it would start to fall apart. This same situation applies to adrenal patients. Even though we may supply the proper foods, if we supplement their diets with inferior compounds, we will produce inferior results.

When building materials are to be ordered for the house, the builder must determine the intended size of the structure and decide how much of each type of material must be procured so that all the materials needed will be on hand with little or no waste incurred. The wise contractor spends a great deal of time considering the size and building specifications for any house he is about to build. In the same manner, a good clinician must give careful consideration to the treatment and management of his patient. Theoretically, the clinician should be even more thoughtful because a house is only a house, but a person is a human being—a temple of the living God.

Making Correct Choices. How does the clinician make the correct choices? On what does he base his opinion? Using the analogy of the house, one may ask, how do we know what kind of house we are building? How do we know which are the best materials? How do we know how much of each particular material to supply?

The answer must start with the developer. He must conceive an idea of the type of house he wants, then he must consult with various architects until he finds one who will produce plans which properly depict his conception. Next a contractor must be commissioned who will carry out the plans in the manner conceived by the developer and depicted by the architect. At this time the proper materials may be selected and the construction of the structure begun. So it is with the treatment of the Adrenal Syndrome patient who, in the analogy, is the developer.

First, the patient must want to improve his situation, he must have the desire to make the effort necessary to regain his health. The effort should start with the search for the proper physician. This doctor will represent both architect and contractor for the patient. Working with the physician, the patient will rebuild his neuroglandular system.

As a first step, the body must be thoroughly analyzed so that the proper nutritional needs can be determined. This chapter is devoted to explaining new and exciting methods for determining nutritional needs. Before we delve into this subject, however, I wish to return to the house analogy for clarification of an important point. Supplying only the proper foods and nutritional supplements without the various regenerative treatments is the same as merely placing the materials on the building lot. These acts alone will not build the house nor cure the Adrenal Syndrome patient. Merely to supply the materials to build the house without actually hiring carpenters, plumbers, masons, electricians, and so on is the same as supplying the nutritional elements to overcome Adrenal Syndrome without utilizing the Magnatherm, Myoflex, tissue-sludge therapy, chiropractic adjustment, counseling facilities, and other components that are the construction work which rebuild strength and vitality in the patient's neuroglandular system, as described in the foregoing Chapters II and III. Many patients expect to overcome Adrenal Syndrome by the use of nutritional substances alone. This concept is a fallacy. It is as unsupportable as expecting to build a house by the mere acquisition of necessary materials.

So just as the construction of a house requires materials, workmen, and the contractor, and/or architect to oversee the work, so must the Adrenal Syndrome patient have a doctor who carefully balances each part of the patient's therapy so that recovery not only becomes possible but inevitable.

Modern Nutritional Analysis

As a whole, it is much easier for the contractor to supply the proper construction materials than it is for the clinician to determine and prescribe foods and supplements for the Adrenal Syndrome patient. The doctor must ascertain the nutritional and chemical deficiencies and imbalances of the patient, *know* which substances will provide the optimal milieu for correction, and how much of each of the remedies the patient will require. These answers are not easily found. Fortunately, with the advance of computer technology and other improvements in laboratory equipment, we are now capable of analyzing the patient's tissues to discover levels of the elements in the body and, with this information, determine what substances are needed to correct the deficiencies and imbalances.

Before I describe these new methods and techniques in detail, I wish to comment on past and present methods used by many nutritionists. In the beginning of medicine, little was understood about nutritional deficiencies and imbalances, As civilization and medical science advanced, knowledge of this subject began to evolve. Almost invariably, nutritional needs were discovered by the empirical correction of a symptom pattern or disease that had been unresponsive to treatment, such as the use of limes by the English sailors to overcome scurvy, rice polishings to counter beriberi, or niacin-rich foods to cure pellagra. Soon nutritional elements were considered to be on a par with drugs and other medicinal compounds; they were used as a specific medicine to overcome a symptom or disease. We now know that many nutritional elements are needed by the body and that, if the body is to function properly, these must be available and *balanced.* To take vitamins and minerals indiscriminately without knowledge of the exact balance in a given case is to court trouble. To recommend one vitamin for one thing and another for something else is to ignore the need for a balance of vitamins and minerals in the body, for, if any one vitamin is taken in greater than normal amounts for any length of time, it can create relative deficiencies of other nutrients.

The great, early health advocates, such as Adelle Davis, Victor Lindlahr, and J. I. Rodale, recommended one substance for one condition, a second for another ailment, and so on. While all of these recommendations were made in good faith and undoubtedly achieved positive results, this method of prescribing nutritional supplements presents problems. It is difficult for a patient to assess a symptom pattern and reach a diagnosis. For instance, a patient may read that a certain element has given good results in the treatment of arthritis. What has proven helpful for one type of arthritis is not necessarily good for another, and such experimental treatment may actually exacerbate or aggravate his condition. He does know that he experiences aches and pains and that the remedy recommended by the health specialist sounds as if it might help. Perhaps the recommendation will help, perhaps not. It might push the system out of balance even more. Following this practice is akin to walking into a drug store and asking the pharmacist for a prescription to alleviate a painful symptom. The pharmacist should recommend that the customer consult a physician to diagnose and treat the condition properly. Were the pharmacist to say, "Sure, try this. This helped Sally Jones who had a pain in the same area a few weeks ago," he would definitely be out of line. This analogy is no more ridiculous than taking nutritional substances which purportedly aided someone else with similar complaints.

Indications and contraindications for use of nutritional substances in the treatment of disorders are just as specific as the indications for the use of drugs or other medications. Admittedly, most nutritional preparations are not harmful when used in small amounts. But when nutritional substances are used in large amounts, such as are usually prescribed for therapeutic purposes, results can be disastrous if not used wisely.

While the pioneering work of the early nutritionists is laudable, attempting to apply their recommendations to health problems without first having the body mechanism thoroughly analyzed to ascertain *actual needs or deficiencies* does their memory and one's self a distinct disservice. Most lay people are not only prone to take the wrong element for the treatment of a condition, but they have no real idea of their own body's requirements. For example, if ten patients from our Clinic, who had been diagnosed as having osteo-arthritis, were examined thoroughly for nutritional imbalances and deficiencies, almost invariably each would have needs different from the other nine. Therefore, a different nutritional program would be required for the proper correction of each disease state. Not only has a patient a disease, but a disease exists within a patient. The heredity and environment of each patient is different, and these differences produce a distinct set of nutritional imbalances and deficiencies. Unless these individual imbalances and deficiencies are ascertained and remedied, there is no real chance of long-term correction of the difficulty. The validity of this last statement would not be disputed by any reputable nutritionist or clinician, nor would it be opposed by any of the nutrition pioneers I have mentioned. The reason for the apparent conflict is that at the time these nutritionists reported their observations such methods of chemical analysis were not available and, therefore, it was necessary for them to make general recommendations. I am sure they wholeheartedly believed it was better to give such a recommendation than to omit the subject. I firmly believe that such decisions on their parts were correct at the time.

In any science or art, alert practitioners use the most advanced methods and techniques available to them. That is not to say that they do not wish they had superior methods available, but to wait until such methods are obtainable before imparting to humanity the work and understanding they have would be a great disservice. I shall presently outline advanced techniques for analyzing the nutritional needs of the human body. I am sure that ten years from now these state-of-the-art methods will be considered archaic. Undoubtedly, I will look back on this chapter and smile to myself, but at this moment they are the finest and the most advanced methods known for nutritional analysis of the human body. What's more, they are effective; they give us information that has not been heretofore available and they help physicians cure their patients—which is, as they say in the oft-used cliche, "the bottom line."

Body/Nutritional Analysis. For many years the General Nutritional Profile (GNP) has been the bulwark of our patient analysis procedure at the Clymer Health Clinic. This nutritional analysis, developed at the Clinic, consists of an extensive blood-testing program (we were the first clinic to use as a routine part of our blood-screening tests lipoprotein electrophoresis, to measure fat levels; T-4 (Total Thyroxin), for thyroid function; ASO (Anti-Streptolysin O) titer, to monitor or check for an infective condition; and RA (Rheumatoid factor) latex, to test susceptibility to rheumatoid arthritis), a tissue test for twenty-one minerals (toxic and nontoxic), a blood test for the twelve most common vitamins, a comprehensive diet analysis, hair analysis, and a complete urinalysis. The GNP is an exceptionally good diagnostic tool, which has allowed us to recommend thousands of nutritional programs designed for the needs of the individual patient. From the results of these test procedures, we are able to ascertain what substances an individual patient requires and the amount needed of each to balance the system. The experience of anlyzing thousands of GNP results over many years has enabled us to ascertain which compounds are better absorbed and utilized, and which are of lower quality and, therefore, are not recommended by our Clinic. The science of producing nutritional compounds is still in its infancy. For example, according to representations listed on the labels, several supplement products may seem similar, but in practice some are much more effective than others. In addition, benefits derived from nutritional products vary from patient to patient. For instance, one adrenal substance may help twenty-four out of twenty-five patients, but cause one patient stomach discomfort or fail to bring about the desired improvement. For this patient, changing to another brand often corrects the problem. For these reasons we advise our patients to supplement only with the products we know are of value and can, therefore, recommend. The commodity the patient purchases from the physician is counsel and advice; not to consider and/or act upon the advice is akin to throwing money away.

To make full use of the program, it is essential that patients be retested every six months, until such time that their bodies' chemistries are balanced; then retest is recommended once a year for maintenance purposes. In this manner, we are able to analyze the best approach for handling individual problems, and, also, the most useful methods of correcting recurring problems.

Because the analysis program has revealed certain repeating groups of nutritional deficiencies, we can often diagnose a patient's difficulties from the pattern of the GNP. For instance, there is a GNP pattern for hypoglycemia, one for the various types of diabetes, one for many of the enigmatic mental disorders, as well as one for Adrenal Syndrome.

In the early days of my work I diagnosed Adrenal Syndrome mainly from changes in the postural blood pressure and from patient symptomatology in general. However, now we have discovered a specific pattern of nutritional imbalances in Adrenal Syndrome patients, and, whenever this imbalance manifests, we can, in my opinion, make a definitive diagnosis of Adrenal Syndrome.

We have run into patients who, from all apparent symptomatology, appeared to be Adrenal Syndrome cases, but whose nutritional analysis did not follow the usual pattern. Almost invariably, in these cases, further examination showed that some other condition caused the chronic debilitation. This analysis has been of inestimable value to us, for it has saved our time and the patient from disappointment by allowing us to rapidly find, in most instances, the causes of their condition.

Since our pioneering work with the General Nutritional Profile, other doctors and clinics are utilizing this method of patient analysis. As a humanitarian, I must applaud this development, but as a clinician, I must add a word of caution. The true value of the GNP comes not so much from the test procedure itself as from the experience and skill of the clinicians who use the program. The technical methods involved in this type of program are delicate and complex; it is easy to make mistakes unless the technicians involved are careful and highly motivated.

A Word of Caution. Frequently, companies which offer laboratory services attempt to persuade us to change to their company, assuring us that they offer advantages over services offered by the firms we now patronize. We carefully test the quality of services of each prospective laboratory by submitting various forms of double-blind studies. With hair testing, for instance, we take the hair of one individual, usually a member of our staff, divide it into two or three equal parts, and, after it has been well mixed, send it on different days to one of the new companies, using assumed names. Ideally, all of the tests should report out similarly, because they are parts of the same sample. In the companies we use regularly, the tests do show nearly identical reports. From many of the companies we have tested, even those of high renown and repute, however, the sample readings have come back so entirely different that we have judged their technology valueless, possibly even harmful to patients who may use their facilities. It would be possible to increase certain deficiencies and imbalances if a clinician used the hair or tissue analysis tests of these companies as a basis for his judgments. We often inform the companies of the results of our double-blind studies after we receive their analyses, in the hope that they might improve in the future. In one particularly flagrant case, a hair test laboratory rebutted, telling of all the other doctors who were satisfied with their work, but giving not a word of explanation as to why their reports on the same hair varied so greatly. We follow the same procedures with the laboratories who do blood testing and other analyses.

Admittedly, we are the bane of many nutritional testing companies. However, our patients' happiness and at times their very lives depend on the accuracy of our procedures, and we feel we must do all within our power to insure that these procedures are accurate.

Technology is now available for proper nutritional testing; however, as this method becomes more popular more "fly-by-night" outfits will be entering the field—firms which do not have the experience, skill, or motivation to test accurately and whose procedures can possibly do more harm than good. A patient's best assurance is to seek a reputable clinic which will stand behind the tests. Be especially careful of mail order hair tests and those offered by health food stores. They may have neither the knowledge nor the experience necessary to interpret or test the validity of the report.

Results of nutritional testing which are obtained from these procedures must be looked upon in light of the patient's entire problem, and in light of hundreds and thousands of patients with similar difficulties and imbalances. This knowledge must then be combined to suggest the proper routine for each patient individually. It is not possible for a doctor who does a nutritional test now and then to understand the interplay and correlation of these results with the patient's other needs and requirements. One cannot simply take a tissue analysis test and, finding this mineral high and that mineral low, correct the problem by withdrawing the mineral that is high or supplying the mineral that is low. A mineral may be high or low in a test for many reasons. The mineral may be high, not because the body has too much of it, but because the body is not able to utilize it properly and, therefore, it is being stored in the hair tissues. Although the mineral appears high on a test, it may be one that is desperately needed by the body, but which must be supplied in a readily metabolized form other than that which the body is now receiving.

Merely because a mineral is low in the hair analysis does not mean that the body may not have sufficient amounts of this mineral; usually this is true, but not always. Due to some other imbalance, the hair follicle may not be able to pick up the mineral, so that its amount in the hair could be low but body levels normal. This is common in the case of sodium if potassium is deficient. Sodium and potassium always tend to balance one another, and if the tissues are short in potassium, this usually shows in the hair; but to keep the proper balance, the hair follicle will not pick up more than enough sodium to balance the potassium, and so the sodium level will look low when it really is not. *For these reasons a hair test is only as good as the laboratory which runs it and the clinician who interprets it.*

The value of the GNP, as given at our Clinic, is not necessarily in the numbers that are stated in the returned tests, but in these numbers as judged by our previous knowledge and in comparison with thousands of tests which have been taken previously. The information supplied by the GNP is not the "Word of God." It is simply important information which the doctor must utilize in his nutritional, supplemental, and dietary recommendations. This knowledge more than anything else is the most vital part of the nutritional analysis.

Complete Mineral-Testing Procedure. As advanced and useful as the currently used GNP has been, I have long realized that for the best possible analysis of the nutritional states of our patients something further is required. As previously mentioned, a nutritional component may be high or low in the hair without showing the same fluctuation in the rest of the body. Heretofore, the analysis of the other bodily substances was not technically feasible because of the small amounts of minerals present and therefore the large amount of sample required to make an accurate testing. However, as a result of our constant requests, some of the more responsible tissue analysis firms have finally been able to develop a procedure by which the entire progress of nutritional elements in the body can be followed.

As nutritional substances are utilized, they are first taken from the digestive tract into the blood; from the blood they go to the various tissue repositories where they may be needed for body maintenance and repair; and, finally, those in excess or no longer of value are excreted in the urine. To have a truly accurate and complete analysis of nutritional elements in the body, we should know the state of these elements in the transporting mechanism (the blood), the accumulation of these minerals in the target or tissue elements (hair or fingernails), and which and in what quantities are being excreted in the urine. Such a complex analysis is now available. While the cost of the complete mineral-testing procedure is somewhat higher than the General Nutritional Profile, it has been kept reasonable so that all persons who are truly interested in the needs of their body's nutritional health can avail themselves of this latest in advanced technology.

With the initiation of this complete mineral-testing procedure, many of the honest objections which were raised regarding the hair test analysis have been overcome. Since we now analyze three different parameters of nutritional functioning in the body, our knowledge of this functioning has increased manyfold.

For example, if a certain mineral is normal in the blood, low in the hair, and high in the urine, we can readily assume that a sufficient amount is being taken into the body (because of the normal blood levels), but it is not being absorbed and metabolized by the body correctly (due to the low tissue levels and the high excretion levels). Enough of the element is coming in, but the body is not holding on to it; it is being lost through the urine. We know then that we have to do one of two things: Find a form of this element that the body can more readily use or work to normalize the digestive system of the body so that it can break down properly the type of nutritional source that is now being ingested by the patient. Usually in practice we try to work on both of these factors.

In another example, if a mineral is in normal quantity in the blood, high in the hair, and extremely low in urinary excretions, we now know that sufficient amounts of this element are being taken into the system but that through some defect in metabolism it is being retained in the system and not being properly eliminated. This is common, for instance, with copper. In patients with a certain metabolic defect—often seen in those with Adrenal Syndrome—copper cannot be excreted and accumulates in the system. Dramatic changes in personality can occur in this type of individual because such an elevated copper level can cause mental and emotional symptoms which may border on those of schizophrenia. This condition is treatable through a proper combination of zinc, manganese, and rutin, although it takes some time for recovery from the mental symptoms.

Or, if an element is slightly high in the blood, quite high in the tissues, and is being excreted in fairly large amounts in the urine, the answer is obvious—the patient is taking in far too much of this element and the intake level should be reduced.

On the other hand, if an element is slightly low in the blood, quite low in the hair, and being excreted also at a lower than normal level, we know that there is a definite deficiency in intake of this mineral. In this instance we must supply this mineral to a patient in the best absorbable form available.

This method of analysis is of great value. Undoubtedly in years to come, new and more comprehensive techniques will be developed to give greater knowledge of a patient's nutritional needs. However, this new testing procedure along with those we have performed for many years enables us to provide comprehensive and exacting help to Adrenal Syndrome patients in finding their nutritional imbalances and deficiencies. In the past, this lack has been a weak spot in the treatment of this condition; it should be no longer.

Of all the so-called scientific advances of modern medicine, nutritional analysis is one I believe can truly qualify as an honest and useful aid to humanity. The ancients had emblazoned over their temples, "Man, Know Thyself." This is what we are attempting to do with our teaching. Everyday and in every way we are trying to get to know ourselves better, and with these new methods of nutritional analysis we are closer than ever before.

Summary

The correction of nutritional imbalances and deficiences is an essential part of the treatment of Adrenal Syndrome. To this end, all elements and substances the patient needs should be correctly balanced and deficiencies corrected. Exact amounts of the different substances needed to accomplish this end must be ascertained and the patient should be supplied with the best possible products to accomplish this purpose. To fulfill these aims, the General Nutritional Profile, a complete analysis of the body's nutritional mechanism, developed at the Clymer Health Clinic, is essential. In addition to the profile, a three-way analysis—blood, hair, and urine—of the nutritional state of the body is now available. By the use of this triple nutritional analysis, the clinician can easily pinpoint and differentiate imbalances, deficiences, and over- and under-ingestion—not only to indicate what the patient needs, but to know in what form it must be properly utilized and not misused. Even the finest of all of these tests, however, are of no lasting value unless they are backed up by extensive clinical experience and knowledge in their use and application.

CHAPTER V

Patient and Family Responsibilities

As I indicated in an earlier chapter, few conditions in medicine require of the patient such a large responsibility for recovery as does Adrenal Syndrome. Undoubtedly, this is one of the major reasons it is so ignored; few practitioners are willing to spend the necessary time and effort to program, manage, and constantly encourage these patients so that they are capable of carrying out their own parts of the cure. Only the Adrenal Syndrome patient can obtain ultimate control of the condition. The physician can provide a certain portion of the treatment. His part is necessary and vital, but by itself is not sufficient for the total correction of the ailment. Full recovery from Adrenal Syndrome is possible only if the patient assumes his part of the responsibility. If he does not, all help will be slow, arduous, and incomplete.

If this book succeeds in helping the myriads of patients who suffer Adrenal Syndrome to successfully understand the nature of the condition itself, the book will have fulfilled its purpose. Prior to the issuance of this work, all that was available was the twenty-seven page chapter on stress and hypoadrenalism in *It's Only Natural.* (1) All new Adrenal Syndrome patients in our Clinic were told to read that chapter two or three times before their next appointment. I felt that was the only way they could achieve any semblance of understanding of their situations so that I would be able to help them. This understanding is still an absolute essential for patient care. For current Adrenal Syndrome patients, I, of course, require this text. Whenever they feel depressed or have doubts about their condition, I encourage them to read and reread the exposition of Adrenal Syndrome herein.

Steps in the Patient's Recovery

There are five important steps which the patient must take to help himself in overcoming this condition:

1. The patient must fully understand the character and nature of the problem.
2. The patient must accept the fact that he is a victim of Adrenal

Syndrome; not only must he accept this fact in his mind, but also in his heart and soul, so that he has no doubt at all that this is the problem and that he must face it squarely.

3. The patient must evaluate his entire life-style in light of Adrenal Syndrome.
4. The patient must correct his life-style so that he can produce the amount of stress reduction that is required in his specific case.
5. The patient must realize the necessity of, and embark upon, a program of stress reduction that will continue the rest of his life.

Step 1: Understand the Problem. Everything a patient does in his life—be it work, rest, exercise, sleep, eat, enjoy entertainment, take part in any form of activity—helps either to strengthen or to weaken the adrenal glands. Therefore, it is imperative that the patient know as much as possible about every factor, variation, or nuance that might affect him on the road to recovery. My own work, which extends over a quarter of a century, has been a constant investigation of each and every physical, mental, and emotional facet of life that may, in some way or another, help support or injure the adrenal function. I have placed as many examples of these stresses in this book as possible.

Each bit of understanding and information the patient can glean about his problem increases his chance for a rapid and uncomplicated recovery. If questions and doubts arise, the patient is able to return to this text to search for an answer. If a patient has a thorough understanding of his condition, as presented here, he should meet few situations in his existence which he cannot understand and explain. Doubt, fear, and depression arise more from not understanding the real nature of the condition than from any other single factor of Adrenal Syndrome. If a patient has a set of disturbing symptoms, but knows what bodily function is not operating properly and what has caused the malfunction, together with what he must do to alleviate it, a great amount of stress and worry is prevented, and treatment of the condition can progress unhindered. On the other hand, if a patient is having difficulties which he cannot explain or understand, thoughts start passing through his mind that the difficulty might be this disease or that disease; these fears create stresses which produce more symptoms which lead the patient further down a destructive path and can create a serious setback to the improvement of his condition.

The first step on the road to recovery, therefore, is to understand and comprehend basic adrenal reactions. It is a step ignored by too many patients. A good coach in any endeavor always spends a great deal of time acquainting his student with the so-called "basics" of the game, for he knows that in the long run this knowledge usually means the difference between success and failure. Such instruction is usually dull and those involved are often not eager to follow the program, but it is the only road to real accomplishment. The best advice I can give patients is to return to this text and read and reread it until the fundamental nature of the condition is well understood and its various ramifications become as well known as the letters of the alphabet.

It is not always easy for the Adrenal Syndrome patient to comprehend his condition as readily as a more stable person might, because the nature of Adrenal Syndrome causes mental clouding, poor concentration, and inferior memory retention. Therefore, it is necessary for the Adrenal Syndrome patient to spend much more time going over this knowledge to absorb it, but with persistence he will always succeed.

Step 2: Accept the Condition: Step one, patient understanding and comprehension, is relatively easy to explain to the patient and the instructions for its fulfillment are rarely misunderstood. Unfortunately, this cannot be said of step two: patient acceptance of the condition. This point can present a hurdle that is the most difficult part in the entire treatment of Adrenal Syndrome.

For treatment of Adrenal Syndrome to proceed as quickly and as fully as possible, it is vitally important that the patient direct all his energies toward helping himself to overcome the difficulty. The only way that we can help him marshall these energies is if he is positive about what is wrong with him, if he accepts this fact fully and, therefore, is completely motivated to help the doctor overcome his malady. Unless this can be done, recovery will be unnecessarily slow and probably incomplete. Recovery from Adrenal Syndrome always proceeds in direct proportion to the amount of patient acceptance achieved.

If the above statements are true—as they are—and assuming that the average patient is at least reasonably intelligent, one might readily ask why we have so much trouble obtaining patient acceptance. If this acceptance is essential for the well-being of the patient, why cannot the patient recognize this and do all that is necessary to help the doctor aid him in his recovery from this condition?

To understand the patient's difficulty, let us reconsider the nature of the condition, the nature of the Adrenal Syndrome patient, and the advice of the various physicians the patient may have consulted before us. Most of these patients have been diagnosed as neurotic or just plain lazy. Most have fears that some strange, undiscovered disease is gradually eating away at their vitals. When the symptoms of the condition are under control, it is easy for a patient to be logical and reasonable and accept the possibility that he may have Adrenal Syndrome. However, when in the still of the night some of the more bizarre symptoms of this condition occur, it is extremely easy for fear and apprehension to creep into the patient's consciousness or for words of a physician who once pronounced him emotionally unstable to come vividly to mind. Doubt builds on doubt, and by morning the patient can have himself thoroughly convinced that he is mentally unstable or a victim of some incurable disease.

On the opposite side of the ledger, for individuals whose symptoms are not as severe as some it is difficult to accept the fact that they have a condition as complicated as Adrenal Syndrome, since the early manifestations are relatively mild. They want to believe either that they are only overworked or that all they have is a virus.

Step 3: Evaluate. It is necessary for the Adrenal Syndrome patient to go on a true austerity program as far as the expenditure of his own neuroglandular energies is concerned. As he is able to adjust his life-style to conserve these energies as much as possible, he will be able to rebuild the general adaptive mechanism and pay off his past bodily debts. When these are paid off and the neuroglandular mechanism is brought to a state of optimal functioning for this individual patient, his austerity program, i.e., his life-style, can be liberalized to a maintenance schedule. However, he must be careful that he does not once again overextend himself and produce more debts—the practice which had previously brought him into such a poor state.

All patients ask how much they must adjust their life-styles. The answer is at once simple and immeasurably complex. They must adjust their life-styles sufficiently to produce the necessary stress-reduction on the neuroglandular system to allow it to regenerate. Exactly what this means for an individual patient depends on three factors: First, on the extent of the drain on the neuroglandular system; second, on the present life-style of the patient; and third, on the types of treatment the patient is able to obtain for his condition. After analyzing these three elements, we are able to help the patient in the evaluation of his life-style changes.

For example, the young minister from Pittsburgh, mentioned earlier, obviously was an Adrenal Syndrome patient. His condition had become so severe that he had fainted in the pulpit while delivering a sermon. This reaction occurred because of lowered blood pressure and a deficient amount of oxygen available to the brain. At times he became so weak that he had to spend two or three days flat on his back in bed before he could carry on with his work. He was, however, as are so many Adrenal Syndrome patients, a definite overachiever. As soon as he was able to get out of bed, he was out working on church duties, giving lectures in different parts of the country, attending parishioners, and planning new projects. Since he lived about six hours from our Clinic, it was not possible for him to see us frequently. Every attempt was made to find a physician in his local area who was knowledgeable about Adrenal Syndrome. As reported, those who would accept him as a patient seemed to have little knowledge of Adrenal Syndrome, and those who were knowledgeable refused to accept him as a patient. Since clinical treatment of any significant magnitude seemed out of the question for this patient, a radical change of life-style was essential if improvement was to be obtained. He had to give up as many of his external church duties as possible and delegate wherever possible his internal church duties. Eventually, once he was able to regenerate his system, he could gradually return to his various duties. However, I do not believe that, even under the best circumstances, he should ever return to the full intensity of activities that he fulfilled when I first saw him. Admittedly, such an opinion is not what a patient wants to hear. In fact, this patient has had a difficult time accepting Adrenal Syndrome. Nature has a way of helping truth, however, and once he fainted during church services, he had little choice but to accept the condition.

In a similar case, a patient called on me, describing in great detail all her symptoms, each one of which led to the same conclusion, Adrenal Syndrome. She mentioned that while she wanted to come to our Clinic for treatment, it was going to be difficult for her because she was, at that time, holding down three jobs and was working seven days a week. I remarked that her situation would probably be quite easy to help; all she had to do was to give up at least one of her jobs and use that free time to come to see us at the Clinic. I advised her that, in fact, unless she did, there was probably little that I or anyone could do to help her.

Another patient whom I had been treating for some time, achieved good progress up to a point, but could not progress beyond a certain plateau. Review of her treatment program showed she was receiving all of the remedies, following the proper diet, and getting her proper treatments at the Clinic. Only one thing remained for her to do: Change her life-style sufficiently to reduce stress further because she was, as I had told her, still putting out more energy every week than she was producing and, therefore, creating an ever increasing debt rather than building up a reserve in her energy bank. I learned later that she had been active in certain church activities which, while she enjoyed them, were not an absolutely essential part of her life. She gave up these activities and, within two weeks, started to improve again and has continued that improvement. Eventually, as her neuroglandular mechanism strengthens, she can again include these extra church activities in her life. However, had we not analyzed her life-style and changed it at the time we did, she would undoubtedly still be floundering in her recovery and wondering why she did not make the improvement we had promised her.

Step 4: Reduce Stress. Once the patient has adequately evaluated his life-style, he can correct his way of living and begin the accomplishment of stress reduction. In regard to this point, one is constantly reminded of the familiar biblical phrase, "The spirit is willing, but the flesh is weak." It is one thing for a patient to evaluate his life-style and realize what changes must be made, quite another for him to institute these changes and live up to these changes until proper improvement has been attained. For instance, the young Pittsburgh minister, while obviously aware of the measures necessary for alleviation and correction of his problem, was anything but eager to make those changes and was actually strongly opposed to such changes. Well motivated to work for his ideals and life objectives, he had a strong sense of duty and responsibility to those who were dependent on him. He was willing to make almost any sacrifice except that which would entail a change in his basic life-style. In fact, his resistance was such that he altered his life-style only when his symptoms became so severe that he could not physically continue.

A long-time professional acquaintance of mine, Dr. Henry Linke, often said "The way a patient has lived is what has caused the problem he now has. To help the problem, we must change his life-style. You cannot ultimately do one without the other." Dr. Linke told me that over thirty years ago, and each passing year has reaffirmed the truth of his statement.

These first four points of patient responsibility are interdependent. Before a patient is able to change his life-style, he must understand his condition and, therefore, have a reason to change. People do not make changes without a reason or purpose. Once a patient understands his condition, it is easier to accept the difficulty and realize the only way to overcome it is to make the necessary changes in life-style. He must then, with the aid of his doctor, plan these changes and, again with the help of his doctor, carry out the alterations which are essential to his ultimate recovery.

Step 5: Continue Stress-Reduction Activity. Once changes have been instituted and the patient is on the road to recovery, he must consider establishing within himself a never-ending evaluation of the stresses to which he is exposed. Stress is an integral component of life without which life would be nearly valueless. The various stresses of living prompt us to all forms of activity which produce every known improvement and man-made beauty in the world about us. In some individuals, however, an overabundance of stresses can exhaust the neuroglandular mechanism. Adrenal Syndrome patients must be careful to avoid an abundance of stress; they must shun those stresses which are, by their nature, worthless or useless. We refer to such stresses as worry, anxiety, judgment of others, or paranoic-type fears. These stresses have no redeeming features except that by learning to eliminate them we grow stronger and wiser.

Probably the most common question asked me by those with Adrenal Syndrome is, "Will I ever be normal again?" The answer I give is, "There is no such thing as a 'normal' person. We are all crippled to a lesser or greater degree from birth. We all come into the world with the combined heredity of our mothers' and fathers' ancestors, none of whom were normal and, therefore, there is no way that they can create a totally normal child. Your problem happens to be a weakness in the neuroglandular mechanism. Luckily, it is one which we understand; one which we can control; and, in most cases, one which we can correct. It is necessary, however, for you to live more carefully in regard to the various stresses of life than the so-called average individual, somewhat in the same way that the individual who has inherited a mild diabetic condition must watch his diet so that he does not ingest too much sugar. As long as he watches this factor, he can live a relatively normal life. If you, the Adrenal Syndrome patient, learn to control and moderate the various stresses upon your whole being, you, too, can live a relatively normal life."

When an Adrenal Syndrome patient says he wants to be "normal" he means what he believes is normal. He really does not mean what would be *his* own normal state, but what he sees as normal for some other person or for people in general. If a blind person is sick and we help him get well, he does not expect to see again, he only expects to have the additional ailment corrected. This is not true of most Adrenal Syndrome patients. They want us not only to return them to *their* normal state, but also to make them "see again," *i.e.,* they expect us to help them overcome the neuroglandular weakness which is their congenital due. We attempt to do this, not by returning these patients to normal, but by encouraging them to a state of supernormal. They must work to obtain a greater control over their lives than the average person, for only in this manner will they achieve their desires. My college football team had a one-eyed quarterback who was good enough to become nationally famous. He put forth much greater effort than most to reach his goal, with his disability, since he lacked depth perception. However, he did not bemoan his fate. He persisted and outpaced all his two-eyed competition for the position. So must the Adrenal Syndrome patient. In the last analysis, how productive, creative, or normal a life the Adrenal Syndrome patient lives is entirely up to him. To succeed, he must follow as fully as he can the five tenets laid down in this chapter. He must fully understand his condition, must have a complete acceptance of the condition, must evaluate the stresses upon him and his general life-style, must correct these stresses as necessary, and must be eternally vigilant in evaluating the emotional stresses that may come to him during the rest of his life. He does not need to stay away from all stresses, but all unnecessary stresses should be reduced to a minimum so that his energy can be conserved for those activities and emotional situations which are truly beneficial and productive to him on all planes of his existence.

What Every Family Should Know about the Person with Adrenal Syndrome

Almost without exception, the average family and friends of the Adrenal Syndrome patient unwittingly do everything they can to worsen the condition. The harder they try to be helpful, the more injurious become the results of their efforts. There are several simple reasons for this paradox, the most common being that almost all obvious or so-called "gut" reactions toward the Adrenal Syndrome victim are invariably incorrect. The advice, be it professional or amateur, which would fit most persons with symptoms similar to those displayed by the adrenal case are completely ineffectual and usually detrimental to the progress of the Adrenal Syndrome patient. Unlike the true neurotic or basic nonachiever, the adrenal victim wants nothing more than to be able to do all the things his friends and relatives are extolling him to do. The fact is, he is physically incapable of accomplishing these tasks and will remain so until the basic underlying condition is remedied.

The patient with this problem is usually intelligent, highly motivated, responsible, with a great desire to achieve. The difficulty is that he has neither the glandular nor the nervous strength to carry out these desires and ambitions. The fact can create in him a large and often conflicting group of emotional and personality frustrations. Put yourself in his place for a moment and perhaps you will see the sense of frustration which is produced by this condition. You are an individual of intelligence and character. You have desired to do useful and productive things with your life and yet every time you attempt to do something, you become more and more exhausted. Every attempt at productive activity is met with strange nervous anxieties or, as one patient put it, "agitated depression." The only thing that even remotely seems to help is rest and withdrawal from all the fascinating events of life. You are like an athlete who is trained to run the hundred-yard dash, but who collapses after a few yards each time he attempts to run. Soon you stop trying and wonder if there is any sense in training or in trying to accomplish anything because fatigue, anxiety, and failure have become the essence of your existence. Here, of course, is where your friends and family come to your aid. They entreat you: "Now, come on, don't be lazy. Keep going, keep trying." They tell you: "It's all in your mind. Tell yourself you are going to succeed and you will." You consider that perhaps they are right, and so you try harder. The harder you try, the more you stress your weakened glandular system and the more rapidly you fail. The more admonitions and encouragement of this kind you receive from your family and friends, the more guilt you accumulate when you are not able to accomplish. The greater the guilt, the greater the stress; the greater the stress, the less you can accomplish; the less you accomplish, the more you are admonished; the more you are admonished, the greater the guilt, and so on.

In this fashion, well-meaning friends and family members hasten the development of this disease. In fact, from my many years in treating this condition, I have concluded that the most difficult to resolve and the most prolonged of all stresses imposed on the Adrenal Syndrome patient are those by friends and family who are truly trying to be helpful. The ironic saying comes to mind: "With friends like these, who needs enemies."

I wish in no way to be harsh or unfair to the family and friends of the Adrenal Syndrome patient. These patients are the most misunderstood of all disease victims in America today. How can their loved ones comprehend their problems when not even one in a hundred doctors understands them?

A large part of my time and energy in treating Adrenal Syndrome patients is devoted to counseling their family and close friends.

Oftentimes only by enlisting their help am I able to resolve a difficult case. When properly motivated, no other group of people can have such a beneficial effect on the victims of this condition.

What Family and Friends Can Do

Understand. The foremost effort that friends can make to help these patients is to understand as thoroughly as possible the nature and character of the disease. To accomplish this end, I suggest that they read this text thoroughly, not just once, but two or three times until the words are engraved on their consciousness and the spirit of the work itself becomes a part of their being.

There are times, unfortunately frequent in some cases, when Adrenal Syndrome patients can be nearly insufferable. At such times it requires the consciousness and personality of a saint to live with them. Only if the healthy friend or family member is permeated with an understanding of the nature of the Adrenal Syndrome experience can he develop the compassion and understanding necessary to help his poor friend or relative on the proper path to improvement and recovery. One who would be of help to these individuals must be able to push aside his own feelings and personal needs as much as possible and learn to say and do those things which are most inclined to produce improvement for the sufferer. There are those who are not willing to undertake such a task upon themselves and many divorces and broken relationships occur because of Adrenal Syndrome. Interestingly, most persons with chronic Adrenal Syndrome tend to marry partners with strong adrenals. This can be true even though the marriage takes place long before real adrenal symptoms manifest. In this way, one partner is steadfast when the other becomes erratic. While such a relationship helps to stabilize a marriage, it does present a problem in that it is difficult for the stronger partner to understand the weaknesses of his or her spouse since he or she has not experienced similar symptoms. This chapter is intended to help remedy this misunderstanding.

I am often asked: "How can I develop this understanding and compassion, Doctor, when the patient seems to do everything he can to upset me?" The answer I give in my office consultations is this: "Suppose you get on a bus and are about to put your token in the meter. Someone enters the bus behind you and steps on your foot while something he is carrying hits you in the shin. Your shin hurts and your foot is sore. You turn around in great anger ready to read the riot act to this inconsiderate, clumsy individual. Upon turning around you find that the object which hit your shin was a white cane and that the individual you are now addressing is wearing dark glasses and is obviously blind. What happens to your consternation and anger? Immediately, they are brushed aside by understanding. You step out of the way and say to the individual, 'Oh, I am sorry, was I in your way? Please let me help you to a seat.' Which you do. The shin still hurts, your foot is still sore, but your feelings of anger are entirely dissipated and replaced by those of compassion and helpfulness all due to the fact that you have a different understanding of the incident after seeing the individual. The events have not changed from the first insult to your body, but your comprehension of what caused the events has changed completely, and so has your attitude. Thus, it can and should be with your attitudes toward your Adrenal Syndrome friend. He is, as it were, emotionally and physiologically blind. He is not able to change many of his actions; he does not hurt you or anyone intentionally. He is driven to these acts by pressures so great, so difficult to control that even a seraphim would be sorely tired."

There is a Buddhist saying of which I am often reminded in my treatment of the adrenal case: "To know all is to forgive all." If we knew and understood what goes on inside the mind of the adrenal patient, we should be able to forgive him and work to help him on his path back to a productive existence.

Encouragement. Another important step friends and relatives can take to help the Adrenal Syndrome patient toward his recovery is to encourage him. One of the basic characteristics of this disease, particularly in its chronic form, is that of discouragement and depression. It seems to the adrenal patient that life is without joy or purpose, that there is no help, and that he is destined to remain forever in the anxious morass of despondency and depression in which he finds himself.

Sermons and admonitions do not help him; encouragement does. Friends should let him know that they understand his problem, that they appreciate his suffering; but that with the proper treatment and care he will improve. They should let him know that although he will have ups and downs—for this is the nature of the condition itself—he must not give up but continue his treatment until his efforts are rewarded. There is no end to the value of encouragement for the Adrenal Syndrome patient, no end to the need for constant assurance that he is going to get better. In the early stages of treatment, especially for the patient with the chronic form, he has little else to fortify him. His treatment, of course, is helpful, but in the beginning this is directed toward building basic adrenal support and has little effect on his immediate sense of well-being. In fact, early treatment can make the patient feel more tired than previously because the adrenal is resting in its effort to rebuild itself. Encouragement and hope are the mainstay of help at this time. When friends and relatives ask what they can do to help the new Adrenal Syndrome patient, I reply that there are three things which they should give in full measure: encouragement, encouragement, and more encouragement.

Reinforcement: "Let Thine Eye Be Single." Another vital factor, to which friends can contribute, is *treatment reinforcement*. The Bible says: "Let thine eye be single." To succeed, it is necessary to look in one direction, take one way, use one path. Only by directing all the forces and energies of the patient along one line can he accomplish his goal. This is important in treating all Adrenal Syndrome patients, but absolutely essential in chronic patients. Once I have accepted a patient, I attempt to make my treatment plan as clear as possible to friends and relatives close to the patient, so that they can offer their support for this treatment. At no time should the adrenal patient have the slightest doubt that the treatment he is receiving is anything but the best available. Doubt creates negative thoughts and these thoughts depress the neuroglandular system in such a manner as to make progress difficult.

Because of the lowered blood pressure and, therefore, lowered nutrition and oxygen available to the brain of the Adrenal Syndrome patient, he has difficulty making decisions and discriminating among types of therapy. He is easily lead from one path to another if some outside influence works to move him in that direction. Like all sufferers of chronic diseases, he is hoping for a miracle. There are no miracles in Adrenal Syndrome cases, only specific hard work which eventually succeeds in overcoming the condition.

Once a patient has started on a particular plan of treatment, it is incumbent on true friends to help support him in this plan of treatment. The patient should be entreated to continue the chosen treatment plan.

If friends or relatives have any disagreement or apprehension about the type of treatment the patient is receiving, they should discuss this situation with the doctor, never with the patient. If those close to the patient are in disagreement with the treatment, it might be best for the patient to go to another physician. There is little use in a doctor's going all out to help a patient if his efforts are constantly subverted by the patient's friends and family.

In Adrenal Syndrome treatment, the doctor must work diligently to build the patient's confidence in the therapy and in his, the physician's care. Only in this manner will the patient receive the full value of the treatment given. Anything that family and friends do to disturb this confidence can be injurious to the patient and severely slow recovery. Little of this depreciation of the patient's treatment stems from maliciousness or attempt to hurt the doctor-patient relationship, I realize. Most of it comes from a sincere, but misguided, effort to help the patient. Frequently, friends bring the patient newspaper or magazine articles which discuss problems similar to that from which they think the patient is suffering. Usually, these are about conditions which produce symptoms similar to those of the patient's, but which are not related to the patient's own situation. This type of reading produces in the patient, who is unwise enough to peruse them, a sense of confusion. The patient begins to question his doctor's care and to doubt the benefit of his treatment. This confusion, unless rapidly corrected, may act to eat away at the progress made and prevent future improvement.

I do not wish to intimate that the therapy outlined here is the only possible therapy to help these patients, or that I alone have all the answers for this condition. Patients may be helped in many ways. I have attempted to bring together the best methods I know to form a complete treatment for this most difficult disease. I know that other dedicated doctors also do a good job with these patients, for there are "many ways to skin a cat." However, in skinning a cat, it is best to choose one way and not try two or three simultaneously. Once the patient and his family have chosen a method of therapy, they should stick with it and not confuse the patient by suggesting other doctors or other treatments. Should any treatment not fulfill the doctor's stated goals, the patient has the right to discuss the future with the doctor, and if the prognosis does not seem favorable, that patient may wish to look elsewhere. If the patient or family and/or friends lose confidence in the doctor, another must be sought. While in treatment with any physician, however, the best chance of success is by full faith in his care. Again, "Let thine eye be single."

Consideration of Other Factors. While the foundation of friends' help to adrenal patients is supported by the three great pillars already mentioned—understanding, encouragement, and reinforcement—several other considerations should be mentioned. When a patient's condition is severe enough to require his staying at the Clinic, we usually do all we can to isolate him from adverse influences. Frequently, our main reason for suggesting a patient stay at the Clinic is to remove him from the home environment which aggravates his condition. The patient's efforts to keep in touch with those at home often defeat our treatment plan. The patient sometimes behaves like a narcotic addict in relation to his previous situation. He knows that everytime he contacts "the folks at home," they are likely to say things which can trigger old reactions which are detrimental to his recovery. Yet his connection with family and friends is so strong that he continually contacts them even though it devitalizes him, both physically and emotionally.

I have found two solutions to this situation. First, I often explain to friends and relatives the character and nature of the condition and what they must do to be of valuable service to their loved one's recovery. Usually this explanation is helpful and sometimes works very well, but frequently family members are unwilling to cooperate or are simply incapable of understanding the situation. In these instances, and in cases in which friends or relatives do not come for consultation, we insist that a patient not contact his friends and relatives until the negative contact can be controlled by the patient's improved physical condition and understanding of his emotional stresses and sensitivities. With great reluctance do I impose such a blackout, it being far more advantageous to the patient and to me to have the help and encouragement of those at home, but in many instances I am left with no other alternative.

A Few Precautions. Even when family and friends are understanding, knowledgeable, and sympathetic, they should consider a number of important factors involved with patient contact.

All phone conversations should be brief, preferably not over five minutes. Lengthy phone conversations have a deceptive effect on the mechanism of the Adrenal Syndrome patient and can exhaust much more rapidly than direct conversation.

No more than two or three friends and relatives should visit at one time. Most Adrenal Syndrome patients are adversely affected by crowds, particularly visitors the patient does not know well or for whom he feels he must put on a "front." Even old friends should not stay too long (an hour is sufficient) to prevent a drain on the Adrenal Syndrome patient. These precautions are most important when the patient first enters the Clinic. However, as the patient improves, such precautions may be relaxed. A patient may be set back several days in recovery by a visitation of well-meaning friends who wanted to come and cheer him.

I am often asked by persons who sincerely want to help, "What do we talk about with these patients?" Admittedly, this is a difficult point because some patients are very sensitive. If the conversation centers on the patient and his condition, he might feel he is being patronized. On the other hand, if talk is about the things that are going on at home, he may become depressed and despondent because he wishes he could do these also, but cannot. (Remember, I said that these people are difficult to please.)

A few suggestions may help. First, let the patient talk. Let him tell about the things which are now important to him. What is he finding out about himself and about others? Let him tell about his plans for the future. In other words, take a lead from the patient. If he brings up a subject, discuss it—but watch carefully how he reacts. If he becomes quiet and withdrawn, if his eyes start to look somewhat vague and glassy, he is being exhausted, and it is time to change the subject or, if no improvement occurs with a new subject, time to leave. Visiting a chronic adrenal patient is like having lunch with a tiger. It can be done, but it is challenging and one must constantly be on guard. When the patient's eyes look glassy, it's as if the tiger were swishing his tail; it is time to leave.

Making Decisions. Though difficult, it is necessary for the Adrenal Syndrome patient, at times, to make decisions. To the patient, with his oxygen-poor brain, molehills easily assume the size of mountains. However, certain family affairs sometimes require a decision by the patient. All such situations must be handled with great care and delicacy, for the patient often has difficulty understanding the exact significance of many of these arrangements. He will frequently lean too far to one side or the other. That is, he may worry unnecessarily over a simple, uncomplicated arrangement in an attempt to make decisions which are not necessarily related to or concerned with the basic problem. Or, on the other hand, he may continually ignore an important project which has to be completed within a certain period of time and which requires some decision from him for its completion.

In these situations, the family should explain the situation to his doctor as thoroughly as possible and then abide by the doctor's suggestions as to how to approach the patient. Such instances happen in our Clinic with great regularity and usually, if the patient is approached in a knowledgeable manner, the situation is resolved without great difficulty.

Children. Patients with children present unique problems. When it is necessary to bring a young mother into the Clinic as an inpatient, we must consider what to do with her children. Occasionally an infant is brought into the Clinic with the mother. Most school-age children are left at home, under the care of the father, grandmother, or friends. While I do not believe in separating mother and child, in certain severe forms of Adrenal Syndrome there is no alternative.

Depending on the age of the child, he should be taught as completely as possible the nature of his mother's problem. No fanciful stories should be made up, as these can cause severe problems at a later date. Almost any child, from the age of four up, can be told what is "wrong with Mommy." The condition can be explained in language that a child can at least accept, even though he cannot fully understand. If there is real difficulty toward this end, the doctor should speak with the child. In my practice, I do this repeatedly, and often I am able to enlist better cooperation from the children than I can from many of the adults. Children should know that the Adrenal Syndrome patient needs understanding and encouragement from them as much as from any other family member. A child's words of encouragement can be of great help to a loving mother.

While most of the foregoing discussion applies particularly to severe Adrenal Syndrome cases who come as Clinic inpatients, the same information is helpful for those who remain as outpatients. In some ways, the aid and cooperation of friends and family is even more important in these cases, because while the inpatient's family contact is only intermittent, the outpatient's family contact is constant and, if poor in support and encouragement, the stress produced can be severe and unremitting.

Laws of Vibration. We have spoken in this chapter and elsewhere of the vibratory states that exist around these patients. Perhaps a word of explanation would help to understand more fully what is meant by "vibratory states." By its atomic nature, all life puts out certain emanations which we know as vibrations. They have various effects and purposes, most of which are not necessary to mention here. The human being is no exception to this rule. In fact, since the human body is a heat-producing structure with electromagnetic and chemical reactions going on by the billions every second, it produces a strong vibratory or electromagnetic field about itself. This field is effected by the basic electromagnetic and chemical structure of the body, by foods we eat, by the character of our elimination, by the thoughts we think, by the emotions which are prevalent within us, and even by our future aspirations as they affect the physical, mental, and emotional components of our bodies. We all know people whom we instantly like and feel comfortable with. We also know people who leave us cold or unsettled and whom we would just as soon not see again. In these instances, we are affected by the aggragate of their vibratory forces in conjunction with our own. In the first case, the individual's vibratory forces are such that they reinforce and strengthen our own, while in the second, exactly the opposite effect is produced. This response is particularly strong in those with Adrenal Syndrome. If they are around persons who are understanding and supportive, they can be swept along on this support, and great improvement can be brought about in their cases. If there are persons about the patient whose vibratory elements are antipathetic, the results produced are detrimental and the patient's progress can be impeded by these forces of unsympathetic vibrations. It is not even necessary for those around the patient to communicate disapproval. The mere presence of a person who is not understanding, harmonious, and encouraging can be and usually is, injurious to the patient's progress.

Summary

In a few rules, the best route for family and friends to take to help the Adrenal Syndrome patient are: First, and by far the greatest, be understanding. The more these key people understand the patient's condition, the more they can say and do the correct thing at the correct time. Second, this knowledge must be put to good use in the form of encouragement they give the patient along the way of his long and arduous road to recovery. He needs encouragement in the same way that a woman in love wants to hear the words, "I love you." A woman can never be told "I love you" too often, nor can the Adrenal Syndrome patient or friend be given *too much* encouragement. Even if you have told the patient an hour before that he is going to be all right, tell him again because it is on these words that he must live during an important part of the therapy program. Last, friends should help him keep his eye on his goal; do not let him wander into different pathways. It is easy for him to wander, because his journey is often long and, as on all long journeys, he begins to wonder if he has taken the right road. Let the patient know that he is on the right road and that he must continue on it to the end. If there is any doubt as to any part of his treatment, friends and family should have him speak to his doctor, or do it themselves. Unless the physician has the patient's confidence and the family's cooperation and assistance, recovery from Adrenal Syndrome is almost impossible. The doctor can and must do a great deal in the treatment of these patients; however, he is capable of accomplishing the full task only with the help of the patient's friends and/or relatives and, most important, with the cooperation and efforts of the patient himself. Friends and relatives form an important—even a vital—part of recovery. If they do their task—as the doctor does his and the patient cooperates—there may be complete assurance that the patient will be returned to a vital, productive existence.

CHAPTER VI

Sex and the Adrenal Syndrome Patient

One of the questions I am often asked by Adrenal Syndrome patients and their families is, What about sex? The truth is, a nonproductive sexual life is one of the stress-creating problems I encounter most frequently among persons afflicted with Adrenal Syndrome. Although a cursory description of what I mean by a nonproductive sex life is included here, an in-depth explanation of this subject is given in *Creative Sex* (1). For those interested, I highly recommend that book.

As detailed in *Creative Sex*, three factors must be present for sexual activity to create a beneficial effect on the human organism:

1. There must be a physical exchange of both the male and the female sexual fluids at each coitus. This exchange must be made without chemical substances in the vagina which might be detrimental to the activity or absorption of either the male or the female discharges.

2. There must be strong feelings of love, not lust, nor mere sexual attraction, between the copulating couple, or there can be produced in the sexual fluids of one or the other toxic components which are harmful to the physical and emotional health of both parties.

3. There must be a willingness on the part of both participants to accept full responsibilities for the consequences of their act. They must not only accept the possibility of pregnancy in those individuals who are of the appropriate age bracket, but they must also accept the responsibility for one another. Through the combining of sexual life fluids, they have become one person. The biblical phrase is "the twain shall become one flesh." If these responsibilites are not accepted, then an insidious, almost unconscious form of guilt develops which, in my experience and that of many other dedicated investigators, eats at the core of human neuroglandular integrity, often causing, but always intensifying Adrenal Syndrome.

To these three factors may be added a fourth which, though not a primary requirement for neuroglandular sexual stability, is an added bonus to those who are desirous of deriving the greatest possible benefit from their sexual forces. By special training, it is possible for a couple to use their sexual powers to improve and heal diseases and weaknesses of the body. Admittedly, this procedure is little understood and even less practiced in the modern world, but it is available to all who desire it, and can be a most marvelous adjunct in the regeneration of those who have a weakenend general adaptive mechanism.

To the Christian world which has been taught that the sexual function, per se, was the "original sin," it must seem heresy to consider sex as a beneficial or constructive act. That much of the world still considers sex the "original sin," and wishes it would go away, does not change in the slightest the true nature of sex and its great effect on the human organism for good or evil. Sexual congress, per se, was *not* the original sin. The original sin, and in truth the beginning of all sin, was the *misuse and abuse* of the sexual function. Such misuse and abuse still remains today probably the greatest single cause of disease, misery, and emotional instability in the world.

That sexual abuse has the power to degrade and degenerate is little disputed by most of mankind. The very words "degenerate" and "debauchery" carry with them strong sexual connotations. A lucrative component of organized crime is that which is devoted to supplying degenerate sexual activity to the population, be it in the form of male or female prostitution, pornography, or any other form of licentious sexual activity which might be turned into an unholy dollar. We all are familiar with this side of sex, but is there another, equally potent compensating side?

From our observation of Nature, we notice that none of its inherent forces are good or evil. Only the direction and application of these forces make them either constructive or destructive. The greater and more universal the force, the greater the power it will have wherever it is directed. If it is directed in an evil way, the destruction shall be great. If, on the other hand, it is directed in a constructive manner, the benefit can be as great as the destruction would be harmful.

Sex, as any other force in Nature, is just that—a force, a power, a potentiality. It is the manner of its use which determines whether its effects will be good or injurious. If we acknowledge that it has great potential for degeneration and the destruction of man's physical, emotional, and moral fiber, we must agree that the converse is also true; that properly used and directed, sex has an equally strong potential to uplift and regenerate man's physical, emotional, and moral being.

We have been given many gifts by our Creator, but none is greater than our sexual potential. The use we make of it determines its effect for good or ill upon us and upon those who become a part of our responsibility. If we accept this simple fact of life, it behooves us to learn the laws of our own sexual functioning, to attempt to live according to these laws, and to constantly develop their use for constructive and regenerative purposes. As we do this, we will have conquered one of the greatest problem areas of human life and our days will be long and joyous.

The Three Laws of Constructive Sex

First Law: Exchange. It is an absolutely essential requirement for any sexual, regenerative process that there be an adequate, uncontaminated exchange of male and female secretions during the sexual embrace. It is amazing how often this God-ordained requirement is neglected and/or misunderstood by society as a whole and by physicians in particular. As described in *Creative Sex*, the male and female fluids contain many complex organic substances in addition to the basic reproductive cells. These hormonal and nutrient factors are vital to the integrity of the neuroglandular mechanism of both male and female. They are particularly important to the female, as the male nervous system is, as a whole, less fine and less highly organized than that of the female.

Any form of sexual activity or method of birth control which prevents this proper exchange of fluids on a reasonably regular basis will prove detrimental to any married woman, whether or not she has Adrenal Syndrome. If women who have this condition are sexually aroused, but do not absorb the necessary male fluids vaginally, their neuroglandular systems can experience a devastating shock.

A few moments' reflection will recall to mind that several common forms of birth control and/or sexual activity prevent this necessary physical exchange and can create this neuroglandular havoc. Any form of sexual activity which produces an ejaculation outside the vagina prevents this essential exchange. The use of any type of protective sheath, i.e., condom, prophylactics, rubbers, surrounding the male organ during intercourse also precludes any such exchange. Various forms of chemical suppositories, spermicides, and even the ineffectual but commonly used douche after intercourse are detrimental in either physically removing the health-giving substances or in neutralizing portions of them through the chemical action of the agents themselves.

For those for whom contraception is important, there still remain several effective methods that do not interfere with this exchange. On a purely mechanical level, two of the more modern methods of birth control—the birth control pill and the interuterine device (IUD)—do not interfere with this sexual exchange. Unfortunately, both of these methods have other detrimental effects which may lead the intelligent, conscientious woman to seek other methods of contraception. The pill inclines toward various hormonal imbalances and increases the chance of serious vascular difficulties (2-4). The IUD has a nasty habit of burrowing into the vaginal wall, causing various forms of infection and often necessitating complicated surgical removal (5-6). Recent research has also shown that infection with *Actinomycetes* bacterium is now common in women who leave an IUD in over long periods (7-9). This infection can cause a disagreeable pelvic infection which frequently leads to infertility.

Two other methods which allow successful sexual exchange, but which do not have the adverse systemic effect of the contraceptive pill and the IUD, are the diaphragm and the so-called rhythm method. Admittedly, neither of these is perfect, there being no such thing at this time, but when properly used, they can be effective in contraception control without deterioration of the sexual exchange.

For those whose religion or personal conviction does not forbid it, we generally recommend the use of a properly fitted and utilized diaphragm. By "properly utilized," I refer to the fact that in our Clinic, we suggest that contraceptive jelly be used only on the inside of the diaphragm (that part which goes directly against the cervix) and that a nonspermicidal jelly, such as K-Y,[1] be used for the rim of the diaphragm. In this way, essential fluids do not come in contact with any spermicide and are thereby not chemically altered. Purists will undoubtedly contend that a certain portion of the vaginal wall is covered by the diaphragm and can, therefore, not excrete the feminine fluid nor absorb the masculine fluid, as is required. Admittedly, this is true. Approximately one-third of the vaginal wall is covered in this manner. However, long experience by physicians knowledgeable of the process of sexual regeneration has shown that sufficient secretion and absorption do occur in the remaining two-thirds of the vagina to allow full benefit to be gained from the sexual exchange. The physical and emotional benefits gained by preventing pregnancies which the couple could not adequately support more than offsets any minor fluid deprivation that might come from the use of the diaphragm.

As the couple grows older and the secretions and the absorbing ability begin to diminish, the ability to create leaves, and contraception is no longer necessary. At this time, when such

[1]Prepared by Johnson & Johnson, New Brunswick, New Jersey 08903.

increased surface area is needed most, the wife can once again have the entire vagina available for secretion and absorption.

Those whose conviction does not allow use of the diaphragm must depend on methods which restrict intercourse to times when the egg is not present for fertilization. Many age-old counting techniques have been suggested and other modern methods, such as the use of basal temperatures, help in finding these periods of infertility more accurately than in the past. Such methods are at best difficult and undependable; however, there is certainly no impediment to the proper sexual exchange, and where the religion decrees, or the couple desires no mechanical device, there is no other alternative. Some women are more regular than others and, therefore, much more likely to have success with this method of birth control. If this is religiously or morally the only method open to you, I highly recommend that you consult a physician who is well trained in this subject; follow his advice as closely as possible.

One last subject to be discussed is abstinence. Many newer religious groups advise their adherents that the only practical method of birth control is abstinence. While admittedly this method is effective, it is usually detrimental to the neuroglandular systems of both the male and the female. The laws laid down by God for the use of the sexual function are right use, not abuse or nonuse. For all people, but particularly for those with lowered neuroglandular functioning, the exchange of sexual fluids carried out under the proper circumstances is one of the greatest life-regenerating factors known to mankind. Whether this exchange does not occur because of perverted sexual habits or because of abstinence from sexual activity, the results are the same. Admittedly, the married couple who abstains from sex produces less-harmful moral sin than those who abuse the sex function, yet the effect on the physical component of the body is identical. If there is no exchange of sexual forces, there is no exchange. You cannot make something from nothing. Abstinence is not an answer for those who are married. The benefits of sexual regeneration are available only to those who use the sexual function constructively and productively.

Many may wonder about individuals who never marry or who are divorced or widowed. Are these oft-times well-meaning people kept from the beneficial forces of sexual regeneration? The answer is both yes and no. Yes, in that since they have not accepted the responsibilities of marriage, they have no rights to the benefits of the state. Sexual regeneration is one of the major benefits of accepting the responsibility of a home and family. Any attempt in this field, as in all fields of man's endeavor, to obtain the benefits without assuming the responsibilities would be breaking the Laws of Nature and of God, both of which will punish any and all lawbreakers.

The answer to this question is also "no," however, as these persons are not denied the benefits of sexual regeneration. There is another manner in which those who are single can use the sexual forces for their own constructive and regenerative purposes. This method is described in the book *Creative Sex*, but is of such complexity that it is not practical to repeat this instruction here. However, for those interested, I again recommend this earlier text, or better yet, suggest that those sincerely interested make an appointment at our Clinic for a personal consultation on this matter.

Second Law of Sex: Love. While the first tenet of regenerative sex use is somewhat revolutionary, at least it is easier to explain and understand than the second and third laws. The second law, which insists on love between the two parties who participate in the sexual union, at first may seem to be based on some ancient and unexplained religious dictum or on some romantic fantasy. Actually, neither is the case. The requirement that love be present is based on pragmatic functioning of the human body, and is completely explainable in physical terms.

While the first tenet concentrates on quantitative factors, the second is concerned with qualitative factors. In other words, the first tenet is concerned with the mere physical exchanges of the male and female sexual secretions. We assume that these substances will be beneficial. Unfortunately, this assumption cannot always be made. It is a foregone conclusion among advanced endocrinologists that various secretions of the human body can be altered by the mental and emotional status of the individual, and compounds which under normal circumstances should be beneficial and sustaining can become injurious and toxic if produced in an environment of disturbed human emotion (10-11).

However, it is sufficient to say that if one of the parties to the act of love holds within resentment, envy, hatred, or any other adverse emotional feeling toward the sexual partner, the secretions which that person contributes to the sexual exchange can be detrimental to both parties concerned. While we have not heretofore considered the fact, there is always the possibility that a child may be conceived from such a congress and when such emotional disharmony exists, one must wonder what kind of stability will be built into the life of this child. "A bad tree cannot bear good fruit."

Married Adrenal Syndrome patients often have a variety of problems which may alter the qualitative nature of the sexual fluids involved in exchange. Most frequently, the nature of Adrenal Syndrome itself tends to lessen sexual desire, especially in women. This lack of desire can produce a tendency toward abstinence when it occurs in the man, but when it exists in the woman, it can have various effects on the marriage act. If the woman's husband is kind and understanding, he will not force himself upon her and therefore the result is greatly lessened frequency which tends to produce a physiological withering of the sexual function and, of course, little or no sexual regeneration. In these patients a tremendous force for rebuilding health and overcoming Adrenal Syndrome is therefore neglected.

If the husband is not so thoughtful and tends to force his personal desires on his wife, several consequences may occur. Having no great personal desire for the sexual act, she may merely let him have his way, assuming that this is part of her duty as a wife, but not entering into the spirit or pleasure of the act, not so much because she wouldn't like to, but because she is just too tired to create the necessary initiative. Such negative acceptance produces a low quality of exchange. Other women in this situation may feel that their husbands take advantage of a masculine position and force upon them something in which they really have no interest. Therefore, they build within their hearts a resentment toward their husbands' actions and toward sexual activity as a whole. This resentment prevents them from producing constructive sexual fluids and prevents a proper absorption of the husband's fluids, and so while the physical exchange might take place, the quality or the spirit of the exchange is so poor that it can create a detrimental, rather than a constructive effect on both parties. Often in these instances, especially when the Adrenal Syndrome patient is a young woman, her husband is rapidly turned off by her attitude and either looks elsewhere for a sexual outlet, or the couple retreats into a state of voluntary abstinence, either of which prevents the wife from obtaining any of the benefits of sexual regeneration to help her overcome her problem.

Ideally, the sex life of those with Adrenal Syndrome must be lovingly cultivated. Neither abstinence nor force is the answer. The couple must understand and consider the eccentricities of the Adrenal Syndrome patient, but also practice when and where possible sexual regeneration. As this is done, the Adrenal Syndrome will improve and more frequent sexual regeneration can be instigated. In this, as in most things, "Love conquers ALL."

Third Law: Responsibility. Of all the tenets, the third is the most difficult to delineate and substantiate. This does not reduce its importance, and it is just as important as the others in constructive and creative sexual regeneration.

Man is not merely an animal. He is half God, half animal. This unique combination within one being produces a creature who is physically capable of doing all the heinous acts his mind can create. It also gives him a conscience which can drive him to the extremes of despair and depression over the actions of this uncontrolled, carnal entity within him. Most of us have within us a strong sense of natural justice. Even though our human desires may drive us to commit acts counter to the Laws of God and Nature, we know deep down that we are doing wrong and will condemn ourselves, through the conscience. The guilt which is produced causes a stress which is difficult for the most skilled of counselors and physicians to exculpate. There are human beings who are seemingly without conscience or guilt. Many of these merely hide it from their fellowman, but within them there is a gnawing and burning which allows no true rest. Admittedly, there are those who truly seem without conscience, and who are unaffected by what is right and wrong, what is just and what is unjust, or what is fair and what is unfair. These people cannot be reached. They are outside the mainstream of civilization. We can only protect ourselves and those we love from them. The great majority of people do have a conscience, however, and do feel guilt when they have broken the Laws of God.

To understand this tenet of sexual responsibility, one must first understand God's plan for sexual use and health. The basic plan for man's sexual activity is simple, and all evaluation of such activity must be made in direct comparison with the scenario devised by God. Allegorically, when God created Adam, He looked at him and said, "It is not good for man to be alone," and He forthwith created woman. This was one of God's first acts—that of creating the sexual components of humanity—man and woman. Later He laid down the dictum that these two should join and that the twain, that is the two, should become *one flesh*. The whole act of marriage, but particularly that part of it relative to the sexual exchange, has the capability of making this man and this woman one being, or as the Bible says, "one flesh." They become a single human functioning unit. This is the essence of God's plan, the apogee of one part of the creative function.

Ideally, soon after the awakening of the sexual desires in both the male and the female, God planned that the young man and woman should find one another and join together on a life-long journey in which they would raise a family, establish a home as a training ground for this family, and become a strong, powerful functioning unit that would work for the good, not only for themselves and their family, but for all humanity. They would exercise the sexual desires God gave them without any interference in the sexual exchange or without any attempt to use the sexual organs in any manner which does not allow for proper exchange as described in the first law. They would engage in the sexual embrace only when they felt strong love for one another and would never engage in it when there was anger, jealousy, hatred, or resentment within their hearts. By the nature of their love and honesty, they would assume full responsibility for one another, caring for one another "in sickness and in health, for better or for worse, for richer or for poorer," because they had in truth become one person. As such, "that which God has joined together, let no man put asunder."

This is the God-given ideal of human love, marriage, and sex. The closer a human couple is able to come to this ideal, the better will be the chance of using their sexual functioning for regenerative or healing purposes. The further they deviate from this ideal, the less chance they have of succeeding at sexual regeneration.

Admittedly, in this day and age not too many couples fit into this category of an ideal relationship. However, this in no wise changes the fact that such an ideal relationship can exist, and still be God-ordained as ideal for His human creatures' lives. The fact that it is so rare does not show that God is at fault, but only how far we have deviated from the way He would have us go. In any marriage, the amount of guilt created is inversely proportional to the amount of responsibility which the partners of this relationship are willing to assume. Many people today are living with or having sexual relations with individuals who wish to enjoy the sexual and other advantages of such a relationship but are not willing to take upon themselves the responsibilities of marriage and a family. This weakness of character produces subliminal guilt feelings which are a cancer within the system which can destroy the contentment and emotional stability of either or both parties.

All modern protestations to the contrary, in only one way can a man demonstrate his true commitment to the responsibilities inherent in the beneficial use of the sex act, and that is by legally accepting the responsibilities of marriage. Any other modern sophistry is so much seductive hogwash.

It is an unfortunate human trait that most of us are always looking to obtain something for a price less than its real worth. The price of sexual activity and regeneration is the acceptance of each and every responsibility that may accrue from such an involvement. This includes the responsibilities toward the other person involved, toward the children that may come from such a relationship, plus all the other moral and legal responsibilities inherent in producing a home and family.

Men, particularly, from time immemorial, have done everything within their power to sidestep this responsibility, while still enjoying the pleasures of sex. Only within recent years, however, have they been so seductive in their arguments that they have been capable of convincing women that the unmarried state also has advantages for the fair sex. This must win the prize as the greatest bit of chutzpa ever to take place in the world! It is obviously the greatest job of salesmanship of all time.

I have counseled thousands of individuals who are attempting to live a sexually active life without assuming the God-ordained responsibilities of marriage. I have yet to find one who could even approach the contentment and stability of the sexually regenerate life, lived according to the Laws of God and Nature. Mankind, it seems, will do everything within its power to avoid doing that which is right and just, and, as a consequence, has brought itself to an unprecedented state of weakness and degeneration—physically, mentally, and emotionally.

Creative Sex

I have often been accused of being a harbinger of doom by telling people what was wrong with the sexual activities of modern life and not telling them how to overcome these difficulties. I hope, in part, to overcome this reputation by discussing, as much as I may, how the sexual function may be utilized to help bodily regeneration generally and the Adrenal Syndrome patient in particular.

When the individual, desirous of sexual regeneration, is married, every effort should be made to engage in the sex act at least once a week. Twice a week is to be preferred, if circumstances and the health of both parties allow. Relations more frequent than this are not detrimental unless they are forced and unappreciated by one of the couple.

If contraception is necessary, a diaphragm should be fitted and used according to the method described herein, unless religious tenets preclude its use—in which case, the patient should confer with a physician well versed in the rhythm method of birth control.

Every effort should be made to develop the love between those participating in the sex act, which should not be consummated if there is resentment, jealousy, envy, loathing, hatred, or any other adverse emotion between either of the partners. If such feelings do exist, they should be talked out before the sex act takes place. If they can be resolved and the feelings of love between the two once again established, the sex act may proceed. However, if the adverse feelings between the couple cannot be resolved, the act should be postponed until such a state of love can once again be achieved.

Whenever possible, a person should not get trapped into so-called "relationships" in which all the benefits of marriage are expected with as few of the responsibilities assumed as possible. Such "relationships" are little more than the modern equivalent of the kept mistress with all of the disadvantages of that situation and with very few of its advantages.

The purpose of this instruction is to keep sex from becoming a stress, to prevent it from having a negative effect on Adrenal Syndrome patients. There is, however, a more important and fascinating aspect of the sex function. That is its use as a healing therapy. It can become a treatment method as potent as any we have in overcoming most chronic ailments, including Adrenal Syndrome.

To be used for healing purposes, one must first fulfill the three primary tenets of sexual activity. When these are followed, a person can, during the rest periods of the sexual act and during the period following the conclusion of this act, command his body to direct these infused energies to the healing purpose desired. In the case of Adrenal Syndrome, during the rest periods of the sex act and during that period following the sexual climax, both partners should hold in their minds and hearts this thought, "We are desirous of utilizing as much as possible these energies which we are exchanging during this act of love, to help build and strengthen my body (her body/ his body), to help overcome the weakness in my (her/ his) neuroglandular system." The words obviously do not have to be the same as these, but the thought and spirit should be.

Admittedly, many will scoff at the ability of such a naive procedure to be helpful, but if they only knew the inherent powers in the creative centers of men and women and the power of the human mind to direct the forces within its domain, they would realize that such use of the sexual forces is in full accord with Natural and Divine Law, and that such healing has a power which is not exceeded by any other known to man.

Summary

Although sex may be a major stress for Adrenal Syndrome patients, when the sexual function is used constructively, that stress can be mitigated. Sex can be a constructive force if three basic laws are followed during the sexual union: First, there must be an adequate, uncontaminated exchange of male and female secretions. Second, there must be love between the two persons who participate in the union. Third, there must be responsibility for the consequences of the union. When these three laws are obeyed, a more important aspect of the sexual function may be brought into being—as a healing therapy—which can become a force not exceeded by any other known to man.

CHAPTER VII

Stresses of the Environment — Internal and External

While many of the stresses on the adrenal patient are obvious, many stresses imposed by environmental factors are not easy to ascertain. These stresses include those over which a patient exercises some control as well as those of the environment which are beyond his control. To release a patient from the grip of these stresses requires the physician's entire skill and acumen. Those discussed here can be broken down into four groups:

1. Various infective states that are infrequently recognized.
2. Allergies—particularly to foods and toxic fumes.
3. Chemical toxicities—heavy metal and organic chemicals.
4. Miscellaneous stresses.

Many of these can be considered as diseases in and of themselves, but all of them may complicate an Adrenal Syndrome case and therefore are germane to our subject.

Infective States

The direct connection between infective states and adrenal integrity has been well documented since the earliest research on this mechanism. Dr. Sajous' research contained many references to the adrenal glands and their relationship to infection (1). This relationship may occur both as cause and effect, and it is often difficult to tell which came first—the weakened adrenal or the infection. Dr. Sajous stated that an adult with normally functioning adrenal glands is relatively resistant to infections. On the other hand, my own experience and investigation has shown that infections place a heavy strain on the adrenal glands and can precipitate adrenal exhaustion, either temporarily in acute infections or prolonged as in the case of chronic infections. Therefore, whenever possible, the treatment of infection should be directed to utilize the body's innate defense mechanisms, to strengthen and fortify these mechanisms to prevent recurring infestations.

Probably the closest most people ever come to experiencing the symptoms of the adrenal exhaustive syndrome is during the period following an acute infection. Whenever an infective state triggers the fever-producing mechanism of the body, stress is placed on the adrenal gland system. If the infection is severe or prolonged, the gland may become nearly exhausted by the time the infection is concluded. The exhaustive weakness that frequently follows a case of influenza or a severe cold is merely an instance of exhausted adrenal glands demanding time and rest to regenerate itself.

If the glands are permitted to rest and a person does not return to heavy activity until his full strength returns, the gland can return to normal and no permanent damage is done to the mechanism. However, if he returns to his daily duties before the body has regenerated fully, there are several possibilities for injury, some more or less permanent. First, recovery may be much prolonged; he may not recover fully for several weeks or even months following the infective ailment. Luckily, most people recover eventually, even if they abuse these glands. However, much inefficiency and prolonged weakness could have been prevented if they had allowed their system sufficient time to recuperate following the infective condition.

In many instances, however, the patient is not so lucky. Some of those who may have borderline adrenal insufficiency can be triggered into true Adrenal Syndrome by this abuse.

In the third instance, the gland regenerates to a functioning level, but does not rebuild to its previous state. The person with this condition is able to work and perform his duties as before, but the glands have been left weakened. The next time this person is placed under stress, the adrenal mechanism may give way due to the weakening created by the previous infection. Our case history books are filled with such records. Once this adrenal breakdown occurs, a person requires the same complex treatment as any other Adrenal Syndrome patient.

Specific Infections. In addition to the general infections mentioned above, several specific types of infections are of great importance to the Adrenal Syndrome patient. These fall into various categories.

First, the localized, acute infections. In this category are such complaints as boils, abscesses, streptococcal sore throat, pneumonia, cellulitis, and phlebitis.

Second, acute systemic infections, both bacterial and viral. Here are such conditions as septicemia, childhood disease (measles, chicken pox, or mumps), and other acute systemic viral and bacterial infections.

Third, local, chronic infections, such as vaginal infections, fungus infections of the ear, *Candida albicans* infections, and herpes infections.

Fourth, chronic, systemic infections, a category which, it must be admitted, encroaches upon the third group, since most modern research physicians believe that the basic infection in these instances is system-wide. These chronic infections in this last category can be either of a severe or of a low-grade nature. In our work with the Adrenal Syndrome patient, we are more interested in the low-grade chronic, systemic infections, since they are more likely to go undiagnosed and untreated.

Acute Local Infections. While acute local infections can have adverse effects on the adrenal mechanism, they are usually of a type that readily falls within the expertise of modern orthodox medicine, and today are not considered the cause of adrenal exhaustion as they were in the past. Improved sanitary conditions, the knowledge and use of nutritional compounds, particularly vitamin C, and the judicious use of antibiotics have helped mankind make great strides in overcoming these once-common causes of death. Most are of bacterial origin and whenever they appear, are usually well handled by antibiotic therapy.

In our work as a natural health Clinic, we use antibiotics only when other forms of more natural therapy have not been able to correct an infection. We attempt to stimulate the body's defense mechanism to overcome acute infections. In this technique, the defense mechanism gains strength by honing the process of antibody formation and directing its own forces. All this is accomplished in the same manner that a battalion of soldiers gain skill and wisdom in fighting by becoming seasoned in battle. When antibiotics are given, the body's mechanisms are not required to control the infection, and no true seasoning of this mechanism can occur. Thus, the body's own defense mechanism remains weak and the patient is inclined to "catch" every "bug" that is "going around."

In acute, local infections, whether treated by use of antibiotics or by the natural methods we prefer, the condition is usually quickly overcome and stress on the adrenal glands, though perhaps severe for a short time, is not prolonged and does not tend to cause permanent damage unless the patient does not allow sufficient recovery time after the infection has subsided. The postinfection recovery time required is similar to that described for the common cold or for flu.

The remarks concerning acute, local infective conditions also apply to the acute systemic variety, except for greater emphasis on both trying to let the body do as much of the work as it can and in allowing sufficient time for adrenal recovery following the acute stage of the infection. This can take weeks or months in severe acute systemic infection.[1]

Chronic Infective Conditions. In chronic infective conditions, the local manifestation often is but a rising to the surface of a systemic infection, and, therefore, both local and systemic chronic infections should be handled together.

In the treatment of recalcitrant Adrenal Syndrome patients, the whole area of low-grade chronic infection is fertile soil for investigation. When the adrenal mechanism becomes lowered in efficiency, the body frequently loses its ability to control a group of parasitic organisms which usually abound on its surfaces and membranes. Studies with new electronic microscopes have found throughout the body almost all dangerous bacteria and viruses known to man. Most people, however, have within them an apparent symbiotic relationship that prevents these organisms from becoming injurious to their hosts. The resistance of the body—and when I say resistance I am speaking almost specifically of those mechanisms which are controlled by the adrenal glands—prevents any adverse effect from these uninvited guests. However, as a person's resistance (the adrenal mechanism) becomes less competent, either temporarily or permanently, these parasites are no longer capable of being controlled, and various forms of infective flare-ups occur in the body. In many instances, all that is necessary to control these low-grade infections is the general support of the adrenal mechanism as discussed in this book. However, in the many instances in which the infection has achieved a toehold, this general support is not adequate, and specific measures must be taken to rid the body of the chronic, infective condition.

In handling most of these conditions, antibiotics have little or at best limited use. To understand this, it is necessary to have an understanding of the basic working of the antibiotic. Despite popular opinion, antibiotics do not, per se, kill bacteria. They only prevent them from reproducing. In acute infections, huge numbers of bacteria reproduce at a rapid rate that could be fatal to the system, if not stopped. The antibiotics are used to reduce the bacterial hoards to amounts which the body's defense mechanisms can overcome. Once the level of infection is reduced to a certain point, the antibiotic

[1]The control of acute infections is treated fully in *It's Only Natural* (2), and I recommend that work for those who desire more information on this aspect of natural healing. The only addition I would make here regards the use of interferon for viral infections of all types. Since the introduction of the natural interferon, I use it in all viral cases with encouraging results. I highly recommend it for all for these conditions.

effect is negligible, and only the body's own processes can eliminate the remaining infection.

In most chronic infections, the level of bacterial proliferation remains below that for which antibiotics are effective. If antibiotics are given, the most they can do is to prevent acute exacerbations, but they will not correct the chronic infection. A typical case in point is the use of tetracycline to treat acne. This antibiotic can be used to prevent severe eruptions, but it does not eliminate the chronic infection. In low-grade chronic infections, the residual bacteria, though below the level which are affected by the antibiotics, are still sufficient to cause severe stresses on the adrenal mechanism.

Many chronic infections are of the viral or fungal variety such as the common herpes and the *Candida albicans* infections. Antibiotics have absolutely no effect on these organisms.

It would seem as if the discovery and use of wonder drugs has kept us from grave dangers of severe acute infections, only to leave us with a background of low-grade chronic infections, which are debilitating to vast numbers of our population. This subject of low-grade chronic infection is one which will be investigated for many years to come. In my opinion, many of the present enigmatic chronic diseases for which medicine knows no cause or cure are actually unknown manifestations of known chronic infections, or low-grade chronic infestations of organisms yet to be discovered.

Among the important chronic infections which are understood and are treatable are conditions caused by *Progenitor cryptocides, Candida albicans,* the various herpes viruses, and *Staphylococcus aureus.* One of the most fascinating research projects concerning these low-grade chronic infections is the work of Dr. Virginia Livingston Wheeler and Dr. Eleanor Alexander-Jackson (3-7). These two have for many years worked on a little-known bacterium called *Progenitor cryptocides.* Their research has proven that this agent is present in almost all human beings. Controlled in most of us, it can cause a variety of disease patterns in those who are susceptible. This organism, *Progenitor cryptocides,* is unique in that it is pleomorphic, that is, it has the ability to change its shape and appearance under different circumstances. Therefore, these doctors believe that it is the offending agent in many conditions for which other organisms have been indicted.

This organism is also unique in that it can be observed in the living blood of patients if a proper type of dark-field examination is made. The degree of infestation and response to treatment can be easily and rapidly monitored by this method.

It is essential to be on the lookout for *Progenitor cryptocides* infection in all Adrenal Syndrome patients. The discovery and correction of this type of infection can often make the difference between their improvement and their steady decline.

The patient's history usually reveals if he is infected with *Progenitor cryptocides.* Patients who demonstrate occasional low-grade fevers for which there is no specific known cause, who have unexplained joint aches and pains that resemble what once was called a rheumatism, who have symptoms of fatigue and general lack of energy which do not seem to fit any known pattern, or in whom treatment has proven ineffective should be checked for possible infection with *Progenitor cryptocides.*

In our Clinic, all patients who come for a general examination are given the dark-field investigation of the living blood. If we find by this test a high percentage of cryptocide organisms, urine culture is made. If this is positive, the diagnosis is specific and an autogenus vaccine (one that is made from the patient's own bacteria) is ordered. Experience has shown that while it is essential to support the general adaptive mechanism in these cases, a real cure is not usually possible until the autogenus vaccine (developed and still produced by Doctors Livingston and Jackson) is utilized.

The use of the vaccine has proven a true God-send to a large number of our Clinic patients. It has helped patients overcome many conditions that previously had resisted the best of our work and orthodox medical practices.

While *Progenitor cryptocides* is probably the most important of the low-grade, chronic infections which affect the Adrenal Syndrome patient, there are others which can have devastating effects in specific cases. Among the newest to come to light is that of the fungus infection, *Candida albicans,* previously thought to be only a female vaginal infection. Through the work of C. Orian Truss, M.D., we have become conscious of the fact that *Candida albicans* can become a systemic infection and affect not only women, but also men (8-10). It has, as described by Dr. Truss, the ability to cause a variety of cerebral allergic reactions. It has been known to be sufficiently severe to precipitate suicide. The functioning mechanism is somewhat similar to that of *Progenitor cryptocides* infections, in that the agent is, according to Dr. Truss, in nearly 100 percent of our population. In most, it is held in abeyance by the body's defensive mechanism. If this mechanism becomes lax, as in the case of Adrenal Syndrome, this agent easily becomes more virulent and systemic. Doctors who have researched this agent believe that, since it is present in most vaginas, it is passed on to children, both male and female, during the traverse of the birth canal. Interestingly, symptom patterns which can be produced by this agent closely mimic those of Adrenal Syndrome itself and its frequent companion, hypoglycemia. The cerebral allergies produced by *Candida's* toxicants produce in some people symptoms mimicking various mental derangements. *Candida albicans* infections can often be picked up from the general history of the patient. Any female patient who has had a history of yeast infections, and who demonstrates some of the bizarre symptoms mentioned above, should be investigated for possible systemic *Candida* infection.

In many cases, however, it is difficult to ascertain whether a *Candida* infection is systemic. Perhaps the best differential diagnosis is one using the response to specific therapy. The oral agent used to control *Candida* infections is an antifungal called Nystatin;[2] another trade name is Mycostatin.[3] One might consider Mycostatin or Nystatin as an antibiotic for yeast substances. Fortunately, unlike the bacterial antibiotics, these antifungal drugs have a low incidence of side effects, due to the fact that there are, as far as we know, no beneficial yeasts in the body. Unlike antibiotics which can prevent the reproduction of the beneficial bacteria in our body as well as the nonbeneficial, Mycostatin and Nystatin can affect only the detrimental yeasts.

If a patient is suspected of having systemic *Candida albicans* infection, a short schedule of Mycostatin or Nystatin, usually helps clear up many of the systemic symptoms. If this does occur, we can be safe in assuming that they were caused by the systemic *Candida* because there are no other effects of the antifungal treatment. On the other hand, if the patient does not benefit from a course of Mycostatin or Nystatin, it does not necessarily mean that that patient is not bothered with a systemic *Candida* problem, as some patients do not respond to these drugs. In these cases, we use a specific *Candida* vaccine similar to that used for the *Progenitor cryptocides,* except that this is a general vaccine and not an autogenus one, as in the case of *Progenitor cryptocides.* This vaccine, with or without the antifungal, has proved successful in most cases. Although much remains to be learned about yeast and fungus infections, recent research has focused on the blocking relationship between *Candida* and hormones, showing how *Candida* can impair their function (11-12). As bodily hormones are excreted, they go by nature to a specific receptor site in a specific organ, similar to the way a key fits

[2]Prepared by Lederle Laboratories, Division of American Cyanamid Company, One Cyanamid Plaza, Wayne, New Jersey 07470.

[3]Prepared by E. R. Squibb & Sons, Inc., General Offices, P.O. Box 4000, Princeton, New Jersey 08540.

into a lock. With *Candida* organism, however, it is as if a counterfeit key, a hormone-like substance—such as an estrogen-like or an adrenocorticol-like product—slips into the lock and blocks the reception of the body's own hormones by an organ. Normal hormonal function is impaired. Thus, *Candida albicans* is now recognized as one of the mechanisms by which Adrenal Syndrome can be brought about. Now that a breakthrough has been made and *Candida albicans* is recognized as a source of possible chronic infection, it is hoped that more work will be done in this area.

A diet for *Candida albicans* patients is given in Appendix I.

One of the most common prevailing low-grade infections at the present time is herpes virus 2. There are, of course, various forms of the herpes virus, from the common mouth ulcer or canker sore, the lip lesion, known as a cold sore, to that which forms the nerve infection of shingles. The most important, however, is the venereal form, type 2, which occurs on the genitalia of both male and female. There has been a tremendous increase in this latest form of herpes due to the increased promiscuity of our sexually liberated society. Those who have read *Creative Sex* (13) are undoubtedly familiar with my thoughts on this subject; however, as a physician it is not my duty to moralize, but to do all I can to help my patients live more productive lives, whatever their own moral convictions.

Herpes is a perfect example of that agent which is dependent on the weakness of the general adaptive mechanism of the body. People who have the low-grade systemic herpes 2 infection know all too well that it will manifest if they eat the wrong types of foods, do not get sufficient rest, or abuse themselves physically or emotionally.

It has been my experience that the condition of the herpes is more dependent on the state of the adrenal mechanism than the adrenal mechanism is dependent on the state of the herpes. Herpes, I find, is not a particularly disabling infection to the adrenal mechanism; however, by supporting the adrenal mechanism, patients who have this infection may be helped.

Experience has proven that the herbal remedies, echinacea, myrrh, and thuja—particularly thuja—can be effective in controlling this agent, assuming that the patient is not otherwise dissipating, thereby causing undue strain on his adaptive mechanism.

Sugar also seems to be a sensitizing compound to certain forms of the herpes virus. If a patient, particularly one afflicted with fever blisters or canker sores, consumes too much sugar and an insufficient amount of phosphorus-free calcium, in the form of calcium carbonate, gluconate, or lactate, the mouth ulcers tend to manifest much more frequently.

Recently, research has shown that the amino acid, lysine, tends to counteract the herpes infection, and many authors are now recommending its use as a treatment for these chronic infections (14-15).

Personally, it is against my principles to take one substance, even though it is a natural substance, out of its matrix and give it in larger than normal amounts to the body. I fear it may in turn create other imbalances which could eventually cause greater problems than the one for which it was prescribed. Time may prove me wrong.

Chronic Staphylococcal Infections. The chronic infection *Staphylococcus aureus* is among the most ancient of all known human infections. Usually, this is the infective organism whenever pus is formed. The encouraging thing about staphylococcal infections is that they are generally circumscribed, that is, the body tends to wall them off so that they can be controlled. Because of this, they do not generally spread systemically. The agent may be systemic at times, but the manifestation is usually local and tends to work toward the surface whenever possible. Boils, carbuncles, abscesses, so-called "pimples," and, of course, lesions of acne are all staphylococcal infections. While these infections, like those of herpes, do not seem to have a profound effect on the Adrenal Syndrome patient who may be afflicted with them, they are certainly a stress and should be eliminated if at all possible.

The staphylococcal germ has the ability to quickly build a resistance to various forms of antibiotics. In fact, several years ago we were often accosted with the term, "Hospital Staph," which was the common name of a staphylococcal germ that had lived in the world of antibiotics to such an extent that it built up an immunity to them. Since the heaviest use of antibiotics occurred in hospitals, this was where the germ lived. During this time, hospitals became some of the most dangerous places on earth to inhabit. As a result of better cleanliness and upgraded handling of various types of disease, this situation has been better controlled. However, the staph germ still is far from being conquered by modern, orthodox medicine.

The chronic, systemic form, as is present in cases such as acne, can be controlled by various antibiotics, but cannot be eliminated from the system by these drugs.

Several years ago a substance was developed that has proven useful in controlling or even curing chronic cases of staph infection. The name of this substance is Staphage lysate.[4] Fully described in *It's*

[4]Produced by Delmont Laboratories, Inc., Box AA, Swarthmore, Pennsylvania 19081.

Only Natural, it is mentioned here mainly for completeness. Staphage lysate is a bacteriophage culture which helps to stimulate the body's ability to build what has been called macrophages or scavenger cells, which work to eliminate the chronic staphylococcal infection. Staphage lysate seems to have no known side effects and, for cases in which antibotic therapy has provided only temporary results, has consistently proven successful in our Clinic.

Allergies and Adrenal Syndrome

It is necessary to diagnose and treat an Adrenal Syndrome patient's specific allergy(ies), although such treatment, in the beginning, is only a stop-gap mechanism until the patient's general adaptive system is built up. Only by establishing normal function in this system can the patient be kept truly resistant and free of these allergic sensitivities. Adrenal insufficiency causes allergies, and allergies weaken the adrenals. Therefore, to establish a cure, it is necessary to work from both ends toward the middle. The general adaptive mechanism must be built up to help control the allergies and the allergies must be controlled to reduce the stress on the general adaptive mechanism.

Identifying Food and Other Fixed Allergies. For many years we have realized that many Adrenal Syndrome patients have shown abnormal sensitivities to certain foods. Some of these allergic-like food problems can be detected and corrected by known diagnostic and therapeutic measures. Unfortunately, however, the great majority of them remain an enigma to us. In recent years, the technology to detect these various food sensitivities has advanced greatly. One new method, the cytotoxic test, allows us to take a giant step forward in the treatment of Adrenal Syndrome and many allied conditions (16-18).

Dr. John W. Tintera believed that all allergies and allergic reactions result from a weakening of the adrenal system (19-20). If this is true, and I see little reason to doubt it, it is readily understood why so many Adrenal Syndrome patients have frequent allergic reactions.

The Adrenal Syndrome patient can be sensitive to many allergy-producing substances of which food allergies are the most ignored and undetected. The food allergies with which most people are familiar are those known by doctors as fixed allergies, that is, a substance which always reacts with an individual patient, whenever he comes in contact with this food, no matter how small the amount may be or how long it has been since he last encountered it. For instance, some patients break out whenever they eat tomatoes. The symptomatic reaction is of no great consequence in the diagnosis of the condition. It does not matter whether they get a stomachache, a rash, or merely become dizzy, these are individual reactions to the allergic shock to the system from the ingestion of the food. Most people who have fixed allergies know all too well which substances cause their reactions, for the reactions are usually dramatic and sudden.

As a patient's general adaptive mechanism is supported and strengthened by the procedures discussed in this book, some of the fixed allergies may improve. However, most fixed allergies are well-entrenched in the genetic structure of the patient, and it may not be possible to eliminate them in one lifetime. For comfort, he must stay away from the offending substance. Usually, fixed-food allergies are not a serious problem in the Adrenal Syndrome patient, as abstinence prevents symptoms and therefore stress.

The number of fixed allergies is usually small compared with the number of cyclic allergies, which are more commonly found in these cases. A variable or cyclic allergy is caused by the short-term buildup of antibodies in the system, which are produced to react to a certain substance. They will abate within a few days if this food is not soon repeated. For example, if a person who has a cyclic allergy to milk drinks milk every day, certain antibodies accumulate in the blood, which eventually react with the milk metabolites, also present in the blood. This reaction is usually not as severe as that of a fixed allergy, but is more insidious, often producing what are known as cerebral allergies—toxic substances which affect the brain and produce a milk-stupifying effect on the whole body. This allergy can destroy that sense of well-being so cherished by us all. These antibodies will remain in the blood and the reactions will occur as long as that person continues to drink milk. However, if milk is withheld for four or five days, the antibodies in the blood will abate, for they have a short life span unless reinforced by continual ingestion of the allergic food. After a week, most antibodies will have left the blood, and so, although the person is still sensitive to milk, he could take a small amount without serious trouble. This is the mechanism behind the diet regimen necessary for controlling, and the testing procedure needed to detect, specific cyclic food allergies.

Actually, the cyclic allergy is not a true allergy, but a side effect of the body's attempt at self-protection. It occurs because a weakened digestive system does not break down food particles properly and incompletely digested particles enter the blood stream. The protective mechanism of the blood reacts to them, as it would to any foreign object, by producing antibodies to rid the body of these substances.

The ideal treatment for this condition is one which enables the digestive system to break down foods completely, so they do not enter the blood stream partially digested. Unfortunately, digestive weakness is one of the first products of Adrenal Syndrome. Therefore, it is little wonder that these cyclic allergies are so common in Adrenal Syndrome cases.

In treating the Adrenal Syndrome patient, we must do everything we can to improve the digestive mechanism. In many instances, by the time we see a patient, the problem has been entrenched for many years, and the digestive mechanism is extremely poor. In fact, many patients can no longer digest and metabolize the nutritional substances which are essential to building the general adaptive mechanism. For these patients we must find and reduce the cyclic allergies before the digestion can be improved.

The Cytotoxic Test. The Cytotoxic Food Allergy Test (see Figure 2) is the diagnostic tool of choice for determining cyclic food allergies. With this test a physician can ascertain the specific food sensitivities of the patient and allow him to select a diet which will give the body an opportunity to again begin some semblance of normal function (21). Although the test, devised by Dr. A.P. Black and modified by Dr. William Bryan, has by some been criticized and described as useless and undependable (22, 23), other investigators have found good clinical correlation for the test when used as a basis for elimination and/or rotation of foods in patients with a variety of health problems and in identifying potential food allergens (24-26). Although "false negatives" have been reported in cytotoxic testing,[5] the test has been particularly useful as a screening method in testing large numbers of potential food sensitizers.

In this test, a portion of the patient's blood is incubated with each individual food extract that is being tested, and both are examined under the microscope. On the slide the technician actually sees the food extract attack and destroy the blood cells. The strength of this attack indicates the extent of the antibody production in the blood stream.[5] Usually in the Cytotoxic Food Allergy Test, these reactions

[5]The cytotoxic test is not always identically reproducible because the white blood cell pool is a dynamic pool with constant change. More often than not the white cells are present in the blood stream for very short periods of up to twelve hours. This, in my opinion, explains the discrepancies in reproducibility of the test but does not detract from the validity of the test.

are rated as "slight" (s), "moderate" (m), or "Marked" (M).

From a single 10cc sample of blood, over 200 different foods can be checked for sensitivity reaction. The time involved in performing the examinations is rather lengthy, and most laboratory technicians can test no more than two or three patients in a day.

The first fifty-six substances shown in Figure 2 are always tested, as they are the most common allergens. The other foods are tested if the patient wishes to include them in his diet.

Most patients, especially those with Adrenal Syndrome, are appalled at the number of sensitivities revealed by the cytotoxic test. One patient's cytotoxic test showed that she was sensitive to every food on the chart except a few items which she had never eaten in her entire life. Such test results can be depressing, unless the patient understands exactly how these sensitivities function in the body and what must be done to correct them.

To better understand the results of the cytotoxic test, I shall go through a cytotoxic test report and illustrate how I advise a patient. You will notice in Figure 2 that several foods are circled "s" for slight reaction, a few are labeled "m," one or two are indicated as "M". The rest are "N" or are unmarked. Foods with an "N" are those for which no reaction was noted under the microscope. Foods without marks were not tested on this patient because she had not eaten them. This chart, by the way, is taken from that of an actual patient and is an average cytotoxic test result.

Heading the list are several common foods, almost all of which caused a slight reaction. In fact, a great many of the foods which make up the average diet are listed here as having slight or moderate reactions. Obviously, to remove all these foods from the patient's diet—as we would with a fixed allergy—would leave this individual with practically nothing to eat. Luckily, the mechanism of cyclic food allergies is considerably different from that of fixed allergies and an adequate diet can be recommended, using the test report as a basis.

The patient has forty-one slight reactions, eight moderate reactions, and two marked reactions. The patient who has more than six or seven slight reactions is considered to have improper digestion and food-sensitivity problems. Removal of all foods marked slight from the patient's diet would accomplish only temporary improvement for he would soon become reactive to the new food he would eat. That is exactly what would happen to this patient if he were taken off the reactive foods and put on "N" foods. Simply because a food is checked as nonreactive does not mean that the patient can eat it with impunity. It means only that at the time of the test there were insufficient antibodies in the blood to cause a reaction under the

NAME ______________ DATE __________ REFERRED BY ______________

PLEASE READ DIRECTIONS ON OPPOSITE SIDE OF THIS SHEET BEFORE FILLING IT OUT

N—Negative s—Slight m—Moderate M—Marked AUTO CONTROL

Food Allergen	Reaction
1. Corn	N s m M
Wheat	N s m M
Egg (whole)	N s m M
Gluten	N s m M
Egg White	N s m M
Egg Yolk	N s m M
2. Milk	N s m M
Beef	N s m M
Lamb	N s m M
Casein	N s m M
Lactose	N s m M
3. Pork	N s m M
Chicken	N s m M
Turkey	N s m M
4. Lettuce	N s m M
Potato	N s m M
Tomato	N s m M
5. Apple	N s m M
Banana	N s m M
Grapefruit	N s m M
6. Lemon	N s m M
Orange	N s m M
Yeast (baker's)	N s m M
7. Cheddar Cheese	N s m M
Cottage Cheese	N s m M
Swiss Chesse	N s m M
8. Roquefort Cheese	N s m M
Hops	N s m M
Malt	N s m M
9. Mushroom	N s m M
Barley	N s m M
Cottonseed	N s m M
10. Oat	N s m M
Rice	N s m M
Rye	N s m M
11. Soybean	N s m M
Chocolate	N s m M
Garlic	N s m M
12. Horse Radish	N s m M
Mustard	N s m M
Onion	N s m M
13. Pepper	N s m M
Coffee	N s m M
Tea	N s m M
14. Almond	N s m M
Cashew	N s m M
Coconut	N s m M
15. Peanut	N s m M
Pecan	N s m M
Salmon	N s m M
16. Shrimp	N s m M
Tuna Fish	N s m M
Sugar (beet)	N s m M

Food Allergen	Reaction
17. Sugar (cane)	N s m M
Yeast (brewer's)	N s m M
Tobacco	N s m M
18. Blueberry	N s m M
Canteloupe	N s m M
Cherry	N s m M
19. Apricot	N s m M
Blackberry	N s m M
Cranberry	N s m M
20. Red Currant	N s m M
Date	N s m M
Fig	N s m M
21. Grape	N s m M
Lime	N s m M
Honeydew	N s m M
22. Mango	N s m M
Olive	N s m M
Papaw	N s m M
23. Peach	N s m M
Pear	N s m M
Pineapple	N s m M
24. Prune (plum)	N s m M
Raspberry	N s m M
Quince	N s m M
25. Strawberry	N s m M
Watermelon	N s m M
Artichoke	N s m M
26. Asparagus	N s m M
Avocado	N s m M
Kidney Bean	N s m M
27. Lima Bean	N s m M
Navy Bean	N s m M
String Bean	N s m M
28. Beets	N s m M
Blackeye Peas	N s m M
Broccoli	N s m M
29. Brussels Sprouts	N s m M
Cabbage	N s m M
Carrot	N s m M
30. Cauliflower	N s m M
Celery	N s m M
Cucumber	N s m M
31. Eggplant	N s m M
Endive	N s m M
Kale	N s m M
32. Kohlrabi	N s m M
Leek	N s m M
Lentil	N s m M
33. Okra	N s m M
Papaya	N s m M
Parsley	N s m M
34. Parsnip	N s m M
Peas	N s m M
Pumpkin	N s m M

Food Allergen	Reaction
35. Radish	N s m M
Spinach	N s m M
Squash	N s m M
36. Swiss Chard	N s m M
Sweet Potato	N s m M
Turnip	N s m M
37. Clam	N s m M
Codfish	N s m M
Crab	N s m M
38. Flounder	N s m M
Haddock	N s m M
Halibut	N s m M
39. Herring	N s m M
Lobster	N s m M
Oyster	N s m M
40. Sardine	N s m M
Scallop	N s m M
Liver	N s m M
41. Gelatine	N s m M
Millet	N s m M
Sesame	N s m M
42. Vanilla	N s m M
Salicylate	N s m M
Saccharin	N s m M
43. Filbert	N s m M
Pistachio	N s m M
Brazil Nut	N s m M
44. English Walnut	N s m M
Black Walnut	N s m M
Carob	N s m M
45. Wheat Germ	N s m M
Wheat Bran	N s m M
Buckwheat	N s m M
46 Yogurt	N s m M
Green Pepper	N s m M
MSG (Accent)	N s m M
47 Sunflower Seed	N s m M
Safflower Seed	N s m M
Jerusalem Artichoke	N s m M
48. Fructose	N s m M
Garbanzo Bean	N s m M
Bee Pollen	N s m M
49. Mackerel	N s m M
Alfalfa	N s m M
Kelp	N s m M
50. Goats Milk	N s m M
Mint Mix	N s m M
Cinnamon	N s m M

Figure 2. Cytotoxic Food Allergy Test

microscope. This may occur from two causes: Either the digestive process is able to properly break down that food and, therefore, no antibodies have been produced, or the food has been eaten so infrequently that the antibodies generated have abated. Unless a patient acknowledges that he eats an "N" food frequently, we must assume that it could be reactive and look upon it the same as those marked slight.

The first thing to be learned from the cytotoxic food allergy test is whether the digestive function is adequate. As noted, six or seven slight reactions on the test generally indicate that the patient has poor digestion; six or less slight reactions usually indicate adequate digestion, although it is to the patient's advantage to rotate these reactive foods.

When a patient has a large number of total reactions, more emphasis is placed on the number of reactions than on the actual foods which caused them because the specific reactions merely indicate the foods which the patient has been eating. A patient with this difficulty usually becomes sensitive to most foods which are eaten repeatedly.

All foods which are labeled "marked" in reaction should be eliminated entirely until we are sure that, through therapy, the general adaptive mechanism has been rebuilt to a point that the digestive system can once again digest these foods. Foods that are labeled moderate should be discontinued for at least a month. If the patient especially misses any of these foods, they may be cautiously added to the diet on a trial basis at this time. However, they should not be used more frequently than once a week, and then only in relatively small quantities.

Foods labeled slight should be rotated on a five-day schedule. That is to say, these slightly reactive foods should not be used or taken more often than every fifth day. This five-day hiatus allows for a dispersal of the antibodies in the blood stream. Consider the example in Figure 2. The patient is sensitive to beef, whole egg, milk, and chicken. On Monday the patient could have chicken; on Tuesday he could have milk; on Wednesday, beef; and on Thursday, eggs. He should not have chicken again until Saturday, or milk until Sunday, or beef until Monday, or eggs until Tuesday, thus allowing at least five days before repeating any one slightly reactive food.

Foods marked "N" can be handled in the following manner: If they are foods which the patient eats frequently, he may continue to eat them at the same intervals as he had at the time of the test. If, on the other hand, they are foods which are eaten infrequently, they should not be eaten more often than every fifth day. As mentioned, if a specific food is eaten fairly frequently, and yet is not reactive on the cytotoxic test, the system is probably able to digest it. If an "N" food is seldom used, its antibody levels in the blood stream would be low, because not enough has been ingested to keep the antibody level high. Since sensitivity is not conclusively demonstrated for infrequently eaten foods, it is best not to eat them more often than every fifth day, for then the chances of building up injurious antibodies are minimal.

Although these instructions are somewhat complex, the subject of food-sensitivities and antibody-reaction is complicated. I have tried to simplify it as much as possible and yet keep the instructions sufficiently accurate to be effective.

Patients often ask me how much of these individual foods they may eat at one time. Actually, experts differ on this subject. Many doctors feel that on the day indicated for a specific food, the patient may have as much as he wishes as often as he wishes. Other doctors believe that the amount of antibodies produced is in proportion to the amount of food ingested, and, therefore, recommend that any individual food be kept within fairly reasonable limits. In practice, I have found that a patient must discover limitations for himself. It depends on foods available and how severely the diet is restricted. In general, I advise patients not to overindulge in any one food but not to eat so little that their diet becomes burdensome.

Much of the developmental work with this type of food-allergy testing was done by the psychiatrist, Dr. William Henry Philpott, who worked out a four-day food-rotation diet which takes into consideration specific foods and, also, specific families of foods for which there might be some cross-sensitization in patients (27-28). Our modification of this four-day-rotation plan is included in Appendix I. We find this plan of use to many patients, particularly since it gives information on the food families. Some patients are so sensitive that even though they stay away from a certain food, if they use a food of the same family, they may sustain antibody reactions. This plan need not be slavishly followed. It is presented only as an example of a diet which does allow a five-day hiatus between the use of certain food families and yet offers adequate nutrition and substance.

Other Tests. Other allergies may affect Adrenal Syndrome patients, and tests have been developed to detect most of these. The four tests available to us are provocative testing, the RAST Test (Radio-Allergo-Sorbant-Test), the eliminative-diet method, and skin tests.

Provocative Testing. Sublingual provocative testing, a method made popular by Dr. Marshall Mandell of Norwalk, Connecticut, consists of placing the patient in a contamination-free environment and putting extracts of various substances under the subject's tongue or injecting them into the arm (29-30). The physician then watches for several minutes and notes specific reactions. If reactions occur, the doctor can use a homeopathic dilution of the same substance tested, in an attempt to find a specific desensitizing dose. For example, if a patient is being tested for gasoline fumes, a certain extract containing this substance is placed under the patient's tongue. After a few minutes, if the patient is sensitive to the substance, he starts to display a variety of symptomatic reactions, such as headache, dizziness, sleepiness, numbness, strange sensations in different parts of the body, or any one of the innumerable allergic-type reactions. When these begin to occur, and if it is desired to desensitize the patient from the specific substance, different homeopathic dilutions of the substance are placed on the patient's tongue. When the proper dilution is found, the patient's symptoms disappear almost instantaneously. Apparently, in these cases, the homeopathic medicine has the ability to affect the general adaptive mechanism so as to counteract the specific symptoms of the symptom-causing extract.

This system has certain limitations, some advantages, and several disadvantages. The most important disadvantage is that only a few substances can be tested at a time. It is a time-consuming process which requires a trained professional to observe the patient under the influence of the allergen and select the proper desensitizing dilution. By comparison, results which can be obtained in a single day using the cytotoxic test, could take several weeks or months when using the sublingual procedure. It does, however, pick up FIXED allergies which the cytotoxic test does not.

Perhaps its greatest use, and the use for which we employ it, is to differentiate from among a few substances which are suspected as being troublesome. If we can narrow down possible sensitivity-producing substances to three or four, the provocative method can be very useful.

This test also allows us to develop a specific desensitizing remedy for any substance to which the patient may be sensitive. There can be circumstances in which a patient simply cannot remove himself from an environment to which he is sensitive. With the sublingual provocative test, we are able to discover a desensitizing agent and thus frequently allow the patient to continue in his present employment. The patient would use this agent whenever he comes into contact with the offending substance. None of the other methods of testing has this option.

RAST TEST. The RAST Test, unlike those previously mentioned, is a standard test performed by most large clinical laboratories (31-32). Both the cytotoxic and the RAST tests use blood specimens for testing purposes. The RAST Test can determine fixed-allergy sensitivities while the cytotoxic test discovers cyclic allergies. The RAST Test is one of the few objective tests for fixed allergies. A disadvantage is that only a small number of substances can be tested and the cost for each item is high, compared to the cytotoxic test. The RAST Test does have a place in the treatment of Adrenal Syndrome patients, not as a screening test, but to help differentiate among a few specific substances. The following substances are now being tested by the RAST method: Almonds, barley, brazil nuts, coconut, cod fish, crab, eggs, hazelnuts, milk, oats, peanuts, pecans, rye, shrimp, tea, wheat.[6] Presumably, in time more substances will be added to make this method more useful.

FOOD ELIMINATION DIETS. A useful method of allergy determination is the elimination diet. Many well-known doctors, such as Dr. Arthur L. Kaslow, of Santa Barbara, California, who is famous for his treatment of multiple sclerosis and similar degenerative diseases, believe that this test is the most practical method of allergy determination (33). He and other doctors believe that they eliminated technical error by working directly with the patient's physical response.

The elimination-diet method is usually pursued by placing the patient on a fast for forty-eight hours and then gradually introducing certain foods which are known to be of a low-allergic nature. If there is a reaction as food items are added one by one to the diet, the reactive food is noted and eliminated. In the Kaslow method, which is probably the most advanced, this process is continued until twelve foods which the patient can tolerate without symptomatic difficulties are determined. These twelve foods are then rotated in a fashion somewhat similar to the four-day rotation diet. This pattern is continued until the patient shows improvement. As improvement progresses, other foods are added to the rotation pattern as long as they do not cause an adverse effect on the patient's condition.

The Clymer Medical Clinic is the only East-coast-based clinic

---

[6]This list represents the foods currently included in our RAST profile. Other laboratories may have slight variations, but basically the pattern is the same.

authorized to offer the complete Kaslow treatment for chronic disease. This method of food desensitization through the eliminative diet has been very effective in many cases of multiple sclerosis and other chronic diseases.

Skin Testing. While the older skin patch method of allergy testing has fallen into the background with many doctors because of the development of the newer methods, it has many uses still, especially for inhaled antigens. These include the common pollens, grasses, and some of the reactive chemicals. The skin test is of little value for food testing, as the accuracy level is low in comparison with the methods already described.

Airborne Allergens. The influence of airborne allergens on the Adrenal Syndrome patient must also be considered. Reactions to airborne allergens can be due to various inhaled substances, such as bacteria, molds, house dust, feathers, or pollen. Most of these cannot be eliminated from the environment except by the most drastic measures, such as moving away from an area that may have a high pollen count or having special, expensive equipment installed in the home to keep dust and mold to a minimum. In some cases such measures may be essential to control the allergy, but in most instances supporting the patient's general adaptive mechanism is sufficient to lessen his sensitivity to the allergy.

One item useful in protecting sensitive patients from inhaled allergens is a mask which has proven helpful against inhalants, including common household chemicals and tobacco smoke.[7] The real problem is to convince patients to use it.

Control of individual particulate matter, i.e., bacteria, small dust particles, or pollen, can be maintained by the proper conditioning of the lining mucosa of the nose. This lining contains thousands of little hair-like projections called cilia which are designed to expel any small particulate matter that are harmful to the organism. When working properly, the cilia have an interesting action—they sweep in only one direction. They erect themselves and sweep outward in one motion. On the return motion, instead of sweeping back like a windshield wiper, they become limp and move back slowly, close to the surface of the mucous membrane. In this manner any small particles which might be inhaled and caught by the nasal mucosa are gradually moved to the front of the nares and out by the normal functioning of the cilia.

---

[7]Manufactured by the E.L. Foust Co., 190 Sunnyside, Elmhurst, Illinois 60126.

In many persons who have inhalation allergies, the cilia no longer function properly and, in some cases, may be almost functionless. This is yet another effect caused by a breakdown of the general adaptive mechanism and is most commonly seen in patients with rhinitis, sinusitis, postnasal drip, and so-called allergies. Upon examining the nasal passages of these patients, the doctor finds a shiny, glaring, red surface rather than the pink, velvet-like membrane of the normal mucosa. He sees at once that the surface has become denuded of cilia, and any foreign particulate substance which enters this individual's nares is easily absorbed into the system since there is no mechanism to prevent it. This foreign substance can set off an allergic reaction, thus causing no end of trouble and further breakdown in the general adaptive mechanism. As the nares' cilia become less effective, more allergic substances enter the system which further depress the adaptive mechanism which, due to its general weakness, cannot support the mucosa of the nose, and around and around the cycle goes.

Fortunately, an effective treatment now exists for overcoming this difficulty by which cilia of most nasal-allergy patients are returned to normal function. The treatment consists of two parts: First, patients are put on a low-mucous-forming diet with a special supplement program designed to supply the body with the elements necessary to rebuild the injured mucosa. The supplements contain natural antihistamines and other substances to help control symptoms while the rebuilding process is under way.

The second part of the treatment is a unique method of therapy developed by two young eye-ear-nose-and-throat physicians who, in a truly brilliant move, found a way to use a common household appliance to treat one of science's most baffling conditions (34).

In an experiment to find a method of reactivating the nasal cilia, they discovered that if a normal saline solution is pulsed at a specific frequency over the membranes of the nose, the solution stimulates the cilia to action, cleanses the mucus, and helps regenerate the nasal membranes. While searching for an instrument that could be used to pulse the solution, they came upon the standard tooth-cleaning WaterPik.[8] They designed a special tip for this appliance and tested it on a group of patients. The results were almost universally successful. After perfecting the special tip, which is plugged into the handle of the instrument, they released their discovery to the medical world. While most orthodox physicians find the procedure alien to their

---

[8]Manufactured by Teledyne Water Pik, 1730 East Prospect Street, Fort Collins, Colorado 80573.

normal training and are not inclined to attempt its use, those who have used this appliance have found that it is the most successful instrument yet devised to decongest the nasal membranes and regenerate the cilia. I have seen patients with nasal allergy of many years' standing who have had little relief from other therapies return to a near-normal status within a short time on this therapy.

Chemical Toxicities

Adrenal Syndrome can be adversely affected by many types of toxic substances. These can be divided into two main groups: poisonous substances which are completely alien to the system and have a direct destructive effect on the protoplasmic material of the body and substances which are beneficial in small amounts, but which become toxic to bodily functioning in high concentrations. The first group can be further divided into those which occur naturally and those which are man-made.

All drugs used in earlier medicine were derived from Nature, because man's skill and expertise had not evolved sufficiently to allow him to construct such substances from basic elements. Some of these natural drug substances, such as belladonna and digitalis, and the heavy metals, which will be discussed shortly, are still used today in medicine and can be toxic if not carefully controlled. Fortunately, the Adrenal Syndrome patient is usually free of most of the conditions which require use of these naturally occurring toxic substances. The possibility of drug toxicity should not be overlooked if a patient seems strangely refractive to therapy.

Several common drugs that are detrimental to Adrenal Syndrome are used daily by much of the population. Adrenal Syndrome patients must stop or severely curtail their use of these drugs if they are to improve. Caffeine has a short-term stimulative effect but a long-term exhaustive effect on the adrenals and must be eliminated before any real progress can be made. Not only should coffee, tea, and cocoa be eliminated from the diet, but also such products as Anacin, No-Doze, and all caffeine over-the-counter drugs should be omitted. Nicotine, another naturally occurring substance, is decidedly toxic to the Adrenal Syndrome patient. Therefore, the smoking and/or chewing—which is not a forgotten art in this country—of tobacco is a "no-no" for Adrenal Syndrome patients. These detrimental drugs will be discussed in greater detail later in this chapter.

Foods of the nightshade family (eggplant, peppers, potatoes, tomatoes) have been pointed to as affecting certain arthritic patients adversely. Possibly, because of the alkaloid nature of their components, they may also have a detrimental effect on some cases of Adrenal Syndrome. In my experience, this is not necessarily a strong factor, but it should be considered if the more common stresses in an unresponsive patient have been exhausted.

While the above-mentioned naturally occurring toxic elements are important in the treatment of Adrenal Syndrome, the body at least has a fighting chance to detoxify these substances to a greater or lesser degree, since these compounds are a part of our ecological environment—we were both created by the same God and came from the same evolution. Man-made organic chemicals, however, are another matter entirely. With these, chemical companies have "for better living through chemistry" created a group of environmental poisons which are unique to our sphere, alien to the basic ecology of the body, and, therefore, in many instances, devastatingly toxic. No doubt they constitute an important factor in the general deterioration of our nation's health. There is not a great deal I need to say on this subject, for authors with far greater skill than I have written many books on the problems of these man-made toxic chemicals. Some of these substances, such as DDT and TCP and dioxin, have become so infamous that even our sluggishly moving government bureaucracy finally stepped in to limit or discontinue their use.

The profusion of these man-made toxic substances is so great, their distribution so wide, and their effects on the human organism so ubiquitous and insidious that only rarely are we able to point to a specific patient and say, "Ah, yes, this is the TCP toxicity," or "This is the BHA toxicity." Man-made organic chemical contaminants are not easily detected because their chemistry is changed once they enter the human body. Their effect on the body is also difficult to ascertain because of the complex nature of the body's enzymatic mechanisms and their interplay with the chemical compounds. It is this indistinct relationship between the absorption of these chemical horrors and symptoms of their toxicity which allows this "greatest of all crimes against humanity" to continue. Because their effects are insidious and subtle and because it is difficult to point to any one substance or manufacturer and say that that substance is the culprit, manufacturers of these death-dealing compounds are able to continue their production until the damage created by their substances has become so obvious that all can see and be affected. By this time, great injury has been done. Even then, when one compound is removed, the manufacturers will produce others to take its place which may have even more harmful effects, only to be discovered at a still later time. So on ad infinitum.

There are only two ways to combat these undiscoverable toxicities. The first is to avoid contact with the toxic substances, and the second is to foster an aggressive program to support those mechanisms in the human body which are designed to detoxify, however possible, these destructive compounds. While the man-made chemicals are not within man's ecospace, the adaptive system of his body can, if strong and expertly fortified, provide him with some protection.

At our Clinic, we make an exhaustive examination of our patients' dietary intake and general environmental life patterns, suggesting changes we feel will help remove such organic toxins from their foods and general habitat.

If the toxic situation is severe, we bring the patient into our Clinic and place him in a specially prepared environment which is as free of such toxic contamination as we can make it. At the same time a special program designed to stimulate and regenerate the detoxifying mechanism of his body is begun. Using these methods, we are able to produce results that have astonished and pleased not only the patients and their families, but also their previous physicians.

Of the enormous amount of disease now present in this country due to the toxic effects of these man-made substances only a minute portion is treated as such. Most of these effects are being treated as some form of emotional or psychological disorder for which more such organic chemicals are prescribed in the form of tranquilizing agents and antidepressants. Hardly a day goes by in our Clinic but that we see pitiful patients who have lost control of their nervous system and have constant involuntary muscular contractions due to long-term use of these two types of drugs.

Of all the insidious dangers to which we, as a people, are subjected, this one creates within me the greatest fear. No one knows what the long-term effect of this multiplicity of man-made toxic substances will produce on future generations. Only within the last forty or fifty years have we been able to produce such a plethora of toxic substances. It will take several generations to even begin to understand the effects such a poisoned world can have on people. When the final results are in, those well-meaning scientists who perpetrated this travesty will be long in their graves, but wherever they are, if there is justice in the universe, and I'm sure there is, we can but offer for them this prayer, "Lord, forgive them, for surely they knew not what they did." The damaging effects on humanity of such men as Genghis Khan, Hitler, and Stalin must be looked upon as infinitesimal beside the deadly human destruction of such misguided misanthropes.

By this time you are undoubtedly asking yourselves, "What can I do to prevent such chemical invasion of my own body?" First, read all labels carefully. Accept nothing with any form of additive unless you know the additive to be safe. Practically no man-made additive is safe, no matter what the Food and Drug Administration may say. Absolutely no one knows enough about the chemistry of the body to know what will happen when we ingest a molecular structure that does not occur in nature. All man-made substances which are ingested, applied, or inhaled by the body must be suspect. All forms of aerosols, hair sprays, toothpastes, antiperspirants, preservatives, colorings must be suspect. There is no such thing as an artificial coloring that is not toxic to some degree. One must go out of his way to purchase food and drink which is as close to its natural state as possible, as little processed as possible, and with as few additives as possible.

Any other attitude is self-destructive.

We should work in our communities to reduce environmental poisoning. If each community will control the companies and factories in its own area, then and only then, can we have a clean world. There is no industrial production or process that cannot be carried out safely if the people involved are willing to spend the necessary time, energy, and inventive skill to do so. However, it will not come about unless we, as an outraged public, demand it. One cannot count on the good intentions of business.

No one is more dedicated to the free enterprise system than am I. I am wholly dedicated to the American dream and the principle of self-determination. However, when any company, in the name of free enterprise and in the search for profits, starts polluting the water I drink and the air I breathe, it has overstepped the bounds of its rights and is infringing upon my rights. I have then not only a right, but a duty to myself, to it, and to the country as a whole to see that it ceases this destruction of our environment. It is encumbent upon us all to do what we can to reduce this chemical exposure to an absolute minimum in our lives and in the lives of those we love. It is also important that we become a voice, a conscience, if you will, for our town, our state, our country to work for laws and programs which will help to reduce and eliminate this chemical contamination. The American dream of opportunity also must carry with it the assumption of certain responsibilities. Unless this is done, it is not a dream—it is a nightmare.

Heavy Metal Toxicity. Of all the toxicities that can affect the Adrenal Syndrome patient the toxicity produced by an excess of the heavy metals in the system is probably of greatest significance. Such heavy metals include copper, lead, mercury, cadmium, nickel, aluminum, and arsenic.

Many of the classical philosophers had a concept in which they referred to the "microcosm" and the "macrocosm," the macrocosm being the world and universe at large, and the microcosm, man. According to this philosophy, the microcosm was identical to the macrocosm except it was in miniature form. In their view, man had within him every element and substance which was present in the larger macrocosm; the proportions were also similar in that elements rare on earth were rare in the human body. I am not personally adverse to this concept and feel that even in the case of such heavy metals as mercury, lead, and cadmium, a minute amount may be useful to the human body. When these small amounts are exceeded, however, serious toxic effects are produced in the system.

There is no doubt about this relationship in the case of copper, selenium, and nickel. These elements are vital to the functioning of the human body. Recent research in Mexico and in the United States, for instance, has shown that a common type of heart disease, present in this part of the world, is directly related to selenium deficiency (35). It is also known that elevated selenium causes specific toxic effects. In working with these metallic elements, a tight rope has to be walked to create the proper chemical balances within the body. We need enough, but not too much. If deficiencies occur, certain diseases can ensue; but if excesses occur, toxic effects will be produced that are particularly detrimental to the adrenal patient.

The heavy metal toxins, though not as insidious as the man-made organic chemicals, are an important part of our toxic environment. Fortunately for us, it is possible by the use of tissue analyses to discover these toxicities. Toxic metal poisoning of an acute, massive nature has been known for some time and has been treated by orthodox medical technology. The chronic type of heavy metal toxicity has largely been ignored. However, with the greater perfection of tissue analysis methods available, even the most hide-bound, orthodox medical practitioner can no longer afford to discount such toxic problems—which have become an important part of medicine and are an answer to many present medical enigmas. The patient with unexplained symptoms and difficulties who has not been checked for metal toxicity has not had the best of modern medical diagnosis. He should have such test at his earliest convenience.

Lead. Lead is one of the most common toxic metallic substances with which we deal. Acute lead poisoning may occur in children who eat leaded paint, painters who are daily exposed to this substance, or persons who work in battery factories and other areas where large amounts of lead are utilized. Such massive toxicity is usually detected before the patient comes to us, so we see few of these patients. The best treatment for this condition is EDTA (ethylene diaminetetracetic acid) chelation.

Many chronic lead toxicity cases are found via hair analysis, and as these cases can mimic the symptoms of Adrenal Syndrome, they are of great importance. When an elevated amount of lead is found, we carefully investigate all possible sources of contamination. Where necessary, we make a test of the elements of the patient's environment, such as well water, home-grown fruits and vegetables, and other ingested or inhaled substances which may be unique to this person. Certain brands of bone meal have proven high in lead. It has been my experience that one must look with great diligence for such sources, as often the toxicity comes from the last thing one might suspect.

I shall never forget a patient from an ecologically concerned family who had moved to a mountainous area of Pennsylvania to "get away" from industry and contamination and to raise their own fruits and vegetables. After the family had been in the mountains a while, their health gradually started to deteriorate. Heavy metal analysis of their bodily tissues showed an overabundance of lead. Try as we would, we could not discover the source. Finally, in desperation, we asked the state agriculture department to check the levels of heavy metals in their home-grown fruits and vegetables. The amount of lead in this produce was found to be well above accepted levels. After giving up home-grown fruits and vegetables and following a concentrated detoxification program, the family regained health. To this day we are not absolutely sure of the source of the excessive lead in the home-grown produce, but apparently their garden was located in a position so that as automotive or industrial fumes were blown across their mountaintop, the lead precipitated onto their growing greenery. This example shows the insidiousness of the pollution of our environment.

The program we use to detoxify chronic lead is as follows: The ingestion of cooked beans (one-half cup daily), vitamin E (up to 800 I.U. daily), B-complex, vitamin C (1000 mg three times daily), vitamin A (25,000-50,000 I.U. daily), and the following oral nutritional detoxifying agents: 1) sulfhydryl amino acid-based products (one to three per day, i.e., methionine, cysteine), 2) deodorized, allicin-free garlic preparations (three to six daily), and 3) broad-spectrum fiber products (bran) (three times daily). (See Appendix III for further information about lead toxicity.)

Calcium, zinc, chromium, manganese, and selenium also provide protection. Calcium from nonmilk sources is preferable, however, as milk products can increase lead absorption. The use of distilled water should be considered as long as the essential minerals are replaced during detoxification, with a multimineral preparation, one to two tablets three times daily, i.e., Seromins.[9]

If the condition does not respond to oral medication, as checked by follow-up hair tests, intervenous (EDTA) chelation should be used. In severe cases of lead toxicity, the change in personality after chelation is often dramatic.

Mercury. Mercury, though not as common a contaminant as lead, frequently appears elevated in mineral testing. Such toxicity generally results from the overingestion of tuna or swordfish, but occasionally its cause is cosmetics manufactured with ammoniated mercury. If a patient with high mercury content is placed on a no-tuna diet and the general detoxification regime, as suggested above for lead, his mercury level usually drops to normal in a relatively short time. If he, like myself, is a great fish eater, he should eat the smaller fish, for the smaller the fish, the lower the amount of mercury. In my experience, while no heavy-metal poisoning is without its adverse effects, elevated mercury levels do not seem to produce as severe an effect as do elevations of lead, cadmium, aluminum, and copper. Other sources of mercury toxicity are listed in Appendix III.

Cadmium. Used as a protective covering for metal objects by various industries and in automobile tires as well as in paint, cadmium is a toxic element which has become of greater importance of late. Cigarettes are also a source of cadmium. Most authorities find it difficult to eliminate cadmium as long as a patient is a cigarette smoker.

Toxology tests reveal that cadmium, microgram for microgram, is far more toxic than lead. Therefore, in elevated cadmium, every effort should be made to find and eliminate, if possible, the source—these sources, along with some of the toxic effects of cadmium, are given in Appendix III.

Aluminum. Aluminum is another common toxic mineral. The main sources, in our experience, are the aluminum chlorhydrate of antiperspirants, the aluminum trisilicate in various antacids, the aluminum salts in double-acting baking powders which are also

---

[9]Prepared by Seroyal Brands, Inc., P.O. Box 6500, Concord, California 94524.

present in most over-the-counter bakery goods, and aluminum cookware. The worst offenders are the antiperspirants. For patients with elevated aluminum levels who use these preparations, we recommend they change to one that does not contain aluminum chlorhydrate. These are available through most health food stores. Read the labels carefully, however; recently a recommended brand has added a new aluminum compound to its formula. Aluminum is aluminum. Beware and reject any product with it, no matter the nature of the compound.

Aluminum is toxic to the brain and the most frequent symptoms of such toxicity are premature senility and loss of memory. These cases are common in our practice; unfortunately, once the memory loss and premature senility have set in, it is difficult to reverse the symptoms. However, stringent elimination of all aluminum sources and a careful detoxification program can do much good in these cases. Nevertheless, it is far better to prevent this toxicity than to cure it.

The treatment of aluminum toxicity is somewhat more difficult than that of some of the other heavy metals. Several researchers have found beneficial effects with the general detoxification regime recommended above plus the addition of homeopathic aluminum in low potencies. (See Appendix III.)

Arsenic and Nickel. Arsenic and nickel are rarely found in elevated amounts in patients. If they are, a careful search must be made for the source, the most usual of which is some form of industrial contamination. Nickel, at times, is found to be high in heavy cigarette smokers. It seems to come from the paper. The cure is obvious. (See also Appendix III.)

Copper. In discussing these toxic metals, I have purposely left copper for last, because its relationship to Adrenal Syndrome is substantially different from that of the other heavy metals. Elevations of the metallic substances previously mentioned cause added stress to the system which must be corrected before a complete resolution of Adrenal Syndrome is to be expected. They are, however, not by their nature directly connected to Adrenal Syndrome. True, elevation of lead and cadmium can cause symptoms which mimic Adrenal Syndrome, but this is basically a problem of differential diagnosis, not one in which there is a direct relationship between the disease and the metal levels. This is not true concerning copper. An elevated copper level often indicates a metabolic defect, which is directly related to Adrenal Syndrome.

The most common hair test pattern observed among Adrenal Syndrome patients is one which presents elevated calcium, copper, and magnesium levels and depressed sodium and potassium levels.

The elevated copper is not essential to this diagnostic pattern, but when it is present, it reveals that the patient has Adrenal Syndrome symptoms and that the elevated copper will complicate treatment. Many researchers feel that the mechanism which creates the weakness in the general adaptive mechanism may also create a fault in the body's ability to eliminate copper and, therefore, it accumulates in the system, creating the problem. This excess copper can create a symptom pattern which parallels that of the hypoadrenal, creating not only tiredness and exhaustion, but also various forms of bizarre mental and emotional reactions. Dr. Carl C. Pfeiffer and his group at the Brain Bio Center, Princeton, New Jersey, found that patients with this condition often exhibited symptoms similar to those of schizophrenic patients (36). Our experience confirms these findings.

There are two types of copper toxicity: that which comes from increased ingestion and that which comes from defective elimination. The first type is not necessarily connected with the Adrenal Syndrome, but the second is. Patients with either type suffer from high copper levels, but the second much more than the first.

In both cases the first essential to treatment is the reduction of copper intake. As far as detoxification treatment is concerned, zinc and manganese, which are antagonistic to copper, are given in large amounts along with a high potency form of rutin, which tends to counteract the adverse effects of copper on the body. These are usually combined with the ingestion of two quarts of distilled water a day for a month to help leech the toxic metal. Such treatment is usually extremely effective, although in certain cases it may have to be continued for several months before it has its required result. (See Appendix III for further information.)

Hair Contamination. Our mineral tests measure elements present in the hair of our patients. It's always possible that the substances we find in the hair may be contaminants and not truly representative of the environment within the body. Especially is this true of the toxic metals. It is Clinic policy to confirm elevated toxic metals found in our hair tests by rechecking with pubic hair. Pubic hair, always or almost always being covered, is usually safe from environmental contamination. About half of our toxic head hair readings prove to be contaminated, as evidenced by comparison with normal pubic hair readings. About the only time pubic hair tests fail is in the prepubic child and in those who swim in pools. These pools, to retard algae growth, use copper sulfate which shows in both pubic and head hair. In both of these instances we take retests with finger- and/or toenails.

Miscellaneous Stresses

There is no end to the catalog of stresses which may affect the Adrenal Syndrome patient. The list is as long and extensive as the imagination of man himself. Certain additional stresses which are not well known, but which have proven to be important causative factors for many Adrenal Syndrome patients, must be mentioned.

Fluorescent Lights. In the light spectrum of most fluorescent lights certain light frequencies are powerfully strong while other frequencies are extremely weak. This produces in a graph of these light frequencies various so-called "spikes," sudden spurts of light energy produced within a narrow frequency range. Experiments, reported in such prestigious magazines as *Scientific American,* demonstrated that abnormal light patterns emitted by fluorescent lights are detrimental to the glandular system of the human being, in particular the pituitary gland. These investigators discovered that many serious health problems may ensue from living or working in an environment of fluorescent lighting (37-39).

The ideal light for man's glandular system, as determined by their research, is daylight. Incandescent light, that is, the regular light bulb, while not equal to daylight, does not have the spikes of the normal fluorescent lighting and, therefore, is not as dangerous as fluorescent lights and can be recommended above them for indoor lighting.

One of the companies that produces fluorescent lights, Duro-Test Corporation, conscious of this problem, has produced a tube known as "Vitalight,"[10] in which every attempt is made to produce a spectrum of light as closely resembling daylight as possible. That they have succeeded may be shown by the fact that their Vitalite can be used as the exclusive light source by which to grow healthy plants.

A patient who is susceptible to Adrenal Syndrome can be severely affected by an environment in which he is exposed to ordinary fluorescent lighting. The best solution for the person who cannot change his employment is to substitute the Vitalite fluorescent tube for an ordinary tube. Almost all patients who have done this have

[10]Manufactured by the Duro-Test Corporation, 2321 Kennedy Boulevard, North Bergen, New Jersey 07047.

reported improvement in their general health and, in particular, freedom from headaches which had often afflicted them.

Alcohol. Alcohol is basically a vasodilator, which tends to open or dilate the blood vessels. In persons afflicted with Adrenal Syndrome, the vascular system is already too dilated by the nature of the disease, and alcohol in any form further aggravates the condition. The Adrenal Syndrome patient, therefore, should abstain from alcohol totally. Not only does it have a direct adverse effect on his neuroglandular condition, but the lack of control precipitated by its effect on the brain centers often leads the patient to activities which produce compounding stresses he would have avoided were it not for the effects of alcohol.

Drugs. Most patients with Adrenal Syndrome have been given various drugs by physicians to help allay symptoms which are part of the syndrome. In the long run, the amount of stress induced in the system by the drug usually far outweighs any symptomatic relief received.

The most common drugs given are the antidepressants and tranquilizers, either separately or combined. In my experience, until the patient is weaned from these drugs, a total cure of Adrenal Syndrome is not possible. However, because of the semiaddictive nature of these compounds, care must be taken in the withdrawal procedure. I have seen cases in which we were unable to discontinue tranquilizers for six months because we had to change the patient's unstable, dependent personality before we dared remove this last crutch.

We find, in our practice, that patients often use any form of stimulus they can to realize some relief from the grinding exhaustion and cerebral dysfunction inherent in Adrenal Syndrome. They guzzle large amounts of coffee, smoke frequently, swallow tranquilizers and mood-elevating drugs in an attempt to give them some semblance of normalcy. Although the effect of these substances is to give temporary succor, they produce a long-term deterioration of the condition and recovery is impossible until they are eliminated. Usually they must be withdrawn one at a time. If a patient is on three crutches, and we remove all three at once, he will fall flat on his face. It has proven most effective to conquer one habit fully before attempting to work on the second and so forth.

Coffee. Coffee drinking, like so many habits which afflict mankind, has created much controversy about its constructive or destructive nature among health authorities. Some consider it a mildly stimulating healthful drink. Others have indicted it as a probable cause of heart attacks and strokes. While there is no consensus of opinion as to the general value of coffee drinking, there is a consensus of opinion as to its effect on the Adrenal Syndrome patient. Because of coffee's short-term stimulating effect, but long-term debilitating and exhausting effect, on the adrenal glands, it is one of the first habits that the Adrenal Syndrome patient must give up if he is to improve. Not only is the caffeine detrimental—since even the decaffeinated variety is injurious to the adrenal patient—but coffee has a specific affinity for the adrenal glands and must be considered the chemical stress par excellence for these patients.

In a patient who uses coffee, alcohol, cigarettes, and anti-depressant-tranquilizer drugs—a surprisingly common combination, by the way—coffee is always the first substance which I suggest be discontinued. Of all of the above-mentioned substances, it has the most direct and profound effect on the adrenal mechanism.

For those who feel that they must have some form of hot drink to take its place, we recommend the cereal "coffees." The ideal substitute, however, is a brew made from *licorice root powder*, obtainable from most health food stores. Properly flavored, this drink is not only tasteful, but contains specific substances which have an extremely beneficial effect on the adrenal glands. When the patient substitutes the licorice root tea for his coffee, fortuitiously he not only manages to give up a harmful habit but also to take on a beneficial one by the same act.

Cigarettes. While few other physicians have mentioned cigarettes, per se, in regard to the adrenal glands, experience has shown that this habit adversely affects the syndrome. Adrenal Syndrome patients who smoke improve only up to a point, and no further, until they are able to give up the tobacco habit. Once they abstain, normal improvement again continues until the condition is resolved.

The pharmacology of cigarette smoking is not as clear or as well documented as that of coffee. It seems to have a somewhat similar effect as this latter substance in that it produces first a short-term stimulation and then a long-term deleterious effect on the adrenal mechanism.

The discontinuance of coffee can produce strong withdrawal symptoms in Adrenal Syndrome patients, but the avoidance of smoking rarely produces these effects. For this reason, I withdraw coffee first, to remove the greatest stress first before I concentrate on the cigarette habit.

Complicating Conditions. Because of the frequency with which a physician encounters Adrenal Syndrome, he must exercise restraint to keep from using this diagnosis too freely. There *are* other conditions which mimic the adrenal symptoms. Many of these conditions may be found in conjunction with Adrenal Syndrome and may require specific treatment before the patient can make the proper progress. Among those are hypothyroidism, myocardial weakness, and B-6 metabolism deficiency.

Hypothyroidism. The lowered thyroid function is frequently induced by the weakened adrenal. This tendency is discovered by the screening blood test made at the beginning of the Adrenal Syndrome patient's care. If the physician is still in doubt, the acciliometer and/or the Barnes temperature tests may be made (40).

If these tests demonstrate a thyroid deficiency, a low dose of thyroid gland, either the fresh extract (Proloid)[11] or the dried (Armour),[12] should be tried. If the diagnosis is correct, the patient should notice improvement in a week or two.

Myocardial Weakness. Another condition which can be an added stress to Adrenal Syndrome, or a condition by itself, is mild myocardial weakness. The weakness of the heart muscle, or myocardium, may be such that it is not sufficient to cause the classic symptoms of congestive heart disease, such as shortness of breath, edema of the extremities, and severe exhaustion, but is sufficient to cause a lessening of the body's efficiency, mild states of exhaustion, and other symptoms which may closely mimic those of Adrenal Syndrome.

While the more severe of these patients can be detected by careful analysis of their electrocardiographs, the EKGs of many of the milder cases do not deviate far from normal; therefore, the milder cases may not surface during a usual examination. In our Clinic, careful analysis of the heart using a sensitive phonocardiograph (an instrument that records the sounds of the heartbeat on a graph rather than the electrical potentials as does the EKG) discloses most of these cases. Weakening muscular contractions of the heart are displayed quite accurately by the phonocardiograph.

Patients with this condition have benefited from using glucoside-rich nontoxic herbs to support the heart action. The best combination

[11]Prepared by Parke-Davis Division, Warner-Lambert, 201 Tabor Road, Morris Plains, New Jersey 07950.

[12]Prepared by Armour Pharmaceutical, Executive Office, 303 South Broadway, Tarrytown, New York 10591.

is a remedy which contains one part Cactus grandiflores to five parts Crataegus oxacanthus. This remedy not only is useful and harmless, even when given over a long period of time, but also has proven to be an excellent tool for the differential diagnosis of this condition. Whenever I have a borderline case, not sure if the heart is involved, I test by giving the proper dose of the Cactus-Crataegus mixture for one month and then discontinue its use for a few weeks. If, during this period, the patient improves in strength and general functioning ability, but then begins to regress a week or two after the discontinuance of the herbal remedy, it is an almost positive sign that he has a minor degree of myocardial weakness.

Since the Cactus-Crataegus mixture is completely nontoxic, and well accepted by the sensitive system of the Adrenal Syndrome patient, if there is any question that an Adrenal Syndrome condition might be complicated by a weakened heart muscle, the Cactus-Crataegus mixture should be used.

B-6 Metabolic Defect. Two recent tests have been added to our repertoire to allow us to measure a new factor in human nutrition: the mauve factor test and the X-K procedure. Both of these tests measure an excess of waste produced because of B-6 deficiency, dependency, or malassimilation. These products are porphyrins in the mauve factor test and xanthurenic acid and kynurenic acid in the X and K test (41, 42). The mauve factor (or kryptopyrrole) often is found in the urine of patients with adrenal dysfunction as well as in patients with mental disorders. Deficiency of vitamin B-6 causes excessive spillage in the urine of the X and K acids which indicates a blockage in the pathway of the conversion of the amino acid triptophane to the neurotransmitter serotonin.

The products of B-6 metabolism are vital to proper brain functioning. If they are deficient, the mind is fuzzy, depressed, and in many ways similar to that encountered in Adrenal Syndrome.

Since we do not as yet know the exact defect in metabolism which causes this unavailability of the B-6 metabolites, we must treat this condition by supplying the end products of this breakdown, pyridoxal-5, phosphate, and L-cystine. When these are supplied, the metabolic defect is circumvented, and the brain once again receives the food it so desperately requires. If this malabsorption has been of long duration, it can take some time before the brain can recover its integrity, but perseverance with the remedies will be rewarded.

It is not known whether Adrenal Syndrome is the cause of this effect, but the frequency with which it is found in these cases is certainly suspicious.

Summary

Many environmental factors create stress in the Adrenal Syndrome patient—factors of which the patient may not be aware. Included are infective states, allergies, chemical toxicities, and miscellaneous stresses. Among specific infections which may have untoward effects on the Adrenal Syndrome patient are acute local and chronic infections, of which *Progenitor cryptocides* and *Candida albicans* can be especially deleterious. Allergic reactions may now be tested in a number of ways, and methods have been devised for protecting against airborne allergens. Heavy metal toxicities may affect Adrenal Syndrome patients—including toxicity to lead, mercury, cadmium, aluminum, arsenic and nickel, and copper. Miscellaneous stresses may be caused by fluorescent lighting, alcohol, coffee, drugs, cigarettes, or by complicating conditions such as hypothyroidism, myocardial weakness, or B-6 metabolic defects.

CHAPTER VIII

A Final Word

There can be little doubt that Adrenal Syndrome is a viable, demonstrable condition. Nor is there doubt in my mind, after detailing its effects for nearly twenty-five years, that the number of its victims increases with each passing day.

Harold E. Buttram, M.D., in his recent book, *Vaccinations and Immune Malfunction* (1), expressed the opinion that one of the major causes of this proliferation may be infant malnutrition and the assault to the immune system by the multiple vaccinations given early in life. If his conclusions are correct, and his logic is difficult to refute, it is hard to explain how any of us escape this energy-sapping problem.

For instance, if a child who may have inherited a tendency toward weak adrenals from his parents, is brought up on the now-popular commercial infant formulas—which are severely deficient in natural food value, the adrenal weakness has little chance to improve. If his already crippled immune system is then assaulted by injection of multiple vaccines into his blood stream bypassing his natural defenses, his immune system is forced to expend much of its reserve vitality to build antibodies for diseases he may never encounter.

By the time this child enters school and is exposed to the multitude of viruses encountered there, he is frequently a ready victim, due to the fact that much of his defense mechanisms have already been committed by the previous vaccines.[1]

[1]As shown in Dr. Buttram's book, *Vaccinations and Immune Malfunction*, according to the one cell-one antigen rule, once an immune body (plasma cell or lymphoctye) becomes committed to a given antigen (vaccine element), it becomes incapable of responding to other antigens or challengers. In the use of the multiple vaccine usually given in childhood, great sections of the immune cells are forced to be committed to the injected antigens (vaccines). These cells can then never be used by the body again to fight any other disease than those now committed. This would not be bad except it has been shown that the vaccination method is extremely wasteful of the immune cells, and many more cells are required to produce immunity from vaccination than are required by natural immunity. It must also be remembered that many of the diseases for which children are vaccinated are not ones usually encountered today. But our antiquated vaccination system, more political than medical, forces the immune system to waste many valuable cells, thereby leaving the child with a lowered defense against the real enemies he will meet.

Should such a child be so lucky as to survive to puberty, the added stresses on his glandular system at this time are usually the final blow to the adrenal. In a real sense he never really becomes a whole person but is crippled by Adrenal Syndrome before he fully becomes an adult.

Unfortunately, this history is not theoretical. It is the exact story I have heard from thousands of patients. Once this scenario has been enacted it can be reversed, but only by great efforts on the parts of the doctor and the patient as described fully in this work.

Adrenal Syndrome is no myth. It is one of the more common consequences of our modern unnatural life. Too long have we as a society assumed that we could abuse the fiats of Nature and God without feeling the result of our disobedience.

Our bodies contain marvelous systems for repair and protection, but unless we wake up and learn to respect and husband them, we will soon find that it is not as now a large minority who has Adrenal Syndrome, but the majority. Should we allow this to happen, we as a nation would fall easy prey to those peoples who, like the Huns of old, have followed the more natural laws of life.

Appendixes

APPENDIX I:

Diets for Adrenal Syndrome Patients

Basic Maintenance Diet

(For those without concurrent hypoglycemia)

This diet, if followed faithfully, will aid in restoring health where lost, and in continuing good health in those so blessed.

First thing upon arising take a full glass of warm water with a pinch of sea salt added. Half a lemon may also be added if troubled with constipation. One half hour later breakfast is taken. Salt may be omitted for persons on a low-sodium diet.

Breakfast #1

Only fruit is taken. One may use as much as desired. The following are particularly recommended: Apples (juice, raw, baked, or as sauce), apricots, bananas (very ripe), berries of all kinds (best raw), cantalopes, cherries, grapefruit (Indian River brand best)*, grapes, lemons*, limes, oranges*, papayas, peaches, pears, pineapples, coconut (fresh best, drink milk), plums, rhubarb*, tangerines*, melons of all kinds. Dates, prunes, figs, and raisins may be used if they cause no trouble, but they are more sugar than fruit and should be restricted during colds, flu, and so on. All fruit should be well washed and preferably rinsed in one of the products, sold at health food stores, to remove chemical sprays. If at all possible, try to buy fruit from a private party or health-food source so that it is without sprays. One of the following may be added to this breakfast, if desired or felt necessary: Nuts, seeds, lean fish or meat. These supply sustenance to the meal without disturbing the digestion.

---

*These foods should not be used if you have arthritis, bursitis, or related diseases.

Breakfast #2 (Nonfruit)

Although a fruit breakfast is recommended, some may find it insufficient at first, or they may wish some diversification. The following may be used in this case:

Cereal: Any whole grain product may be used: Wheatena, steel-cut oats, millet, seven-grain cereal, and other such products.

Milk or Cream: Raw milk or cream is preferred. Some may be used on the cereal and the rest drunk. Cereal coffee or herb teas may also be used.

Bread: Whole wheat toast, whole wheat or corn meal muffins, whole wheat waffles, pancakes or cornbread may be used. (Undegerminated cornmeal)

Raw Vegetables: Raw vegetables may be and should be taken with the foods above because they are all acid-forming and raw vegetables are needed to control this condition. Raw celery or carrots are sufficient.

Dinner and Supper

Dinner and supper both have similar construction. One meal, either dinner or supper, as the case may be, will be smaller than the other, but the types of foods used are not altered, only the amounts.

Protein

Provide *only one protein* at each meal. (Small portions of two proteins from the same group may be used.) Proper proteins may be chosen from the following:

Group I Dairy Products: Milk (raw), buttermilk, home made ice cream. Cottage and natural cheese (no processed cheese), eggs (fertile if possible) soft boiled, scrambed, or raw. (If you have problems with congestion, use only the yolk.)

Group II Meat or Fish: Lean beef, lamb, chicken, turkey, duck, and all organ meats. (If possible, obtain meats from private parties who do not use chemicals in the animal feed or sodium nitrate as a preservative. Some health food stores also carry naturally produced meat.) All forms of fish are good; those from the sea are richer in essential elements than the fresh water fish, however. All types of seafood (clams, shrimp, crab, etc.) are highly recommended as long as their purity of source and processing is assured. Fish and seafood contain less toxic substances than the meats.

Group III Nuts and Legumes: Nuts, lentils, dried peas, beans, and seeds (sunflower, sesame, etc.) may be utilized but with caution, as they are difficult to digest. They must constitute the only starch or protein taken at the meal.

Starches

Have only *one starch* at each meal. More than one leads to overeating. Health-building starches should be chosen from the following:

Whole wheat bread made only from the most natural ingredients. Either make your own or use a whole grain bread from one of the health food stores. A nutritious bread is one of the most important articles of diet; be sure yours is the *best*. Aside from the staple bread, the following carbohydrates are recommended: baked potatoes, natural brown rice, unpearled barley, millet, steel-cut oats, and any products made from natural unrefined grains, i.e., corn bread, whole wheat pancakes, waffles, bran muffins.

Fats

A small amount of fat is useful in most diets. Choose from:

Real butter, soybean-lecithin spreads such as are found in the better health food stores. In cooking only the following products should be used: cold pressed oils, such as peanut, soy, safflower, sunflower, and sesame. For solid shortening, butter or the above soybean spread may be used. These fats may be more expensive than those in usage today, but they may prevent diseases that could cost a thousand times more.

Vegetables

The rest of the meal should consist of vegetables. It is best if they comprise at least one-half the bulk of the meal. This instruction will help to normalize body chemistry. The following comments apply to vegetables: One half of the vegetables should be raw; if you can eat something raw, do not cook it. If at all possible, try to obtain vegetables that have not been sprayed with pesticides or grown with chemical fertilizers. Your best vegetables are those fresh from the garden—yours or a friend's. Canned and/or frozen are allowed, but are second best. Each meal should start with a raw vegetable; this is vital. Tomatoes and/or cucumbers should not be eaten with regular meals, only with other vegetables, meat or fish, not with starches or dairy products.

Additional Instructions

Some products used in preparation of food are necessary but harmful. More healthful substitutes are available and should be used. A list of these follows:

Baking powder: Use only Royal, Rumford, or special health food brands containing no aluminum salts.

Table Salt: Use sea salt from health food stores.

Cornstarch: Arrowroot flour or rice polishings.

Chocolate: Carob candy and powder (El Molino is best).

White sugar, syrups, etc.: Use only turbinado, uncooked honey, sorghum, Grandma's molasses, maple syrup, and maple sugar.

Desserts: Cakes, pies, cookies, etc., can be made from unrefined foods but should be served as the starch for the meal and not afterward, as is usually done.

Coffee, tea: Use the alkaline herb teas, i.e. Alfa-mint, fenugreek, shave grass, clover, rose hips, dandelion coffee, etc.

All foods should be simply prepared. When spices are omitted from the diet, soon the natural flavors of food prevail and our senses can appreciate their delicate but distinctive nature. Natural spices in moderation are not condemned, however.

Do not eat fruit with regular meals, only for breakfast or as a snack between meals and at bedtime.

Nuts, dried legumes, soy beans can be used by those whose digestion allows. They must constitute the only starch or protein taken at a meal.

Do not, under any circumstances, drink fluoridated water or use it in food. Buy bottled water if necessary.

Adrenal Syndrome Diet

(For those with concurrent hypoglycemia)
(Mild, Moderate, Severe)

NOTE: This diet is only a guide; your doctor may not permit some of the listed items.

Upon Arising:	½ grapefruit
Breakfast:	1 egg with or without 2 slices of meat or fish (no ham or bacon) Only ½ slice of bread or toast, with plenty of butter. Beverage (herb tea or cereal coffee)
2 Hours after Breakfast:	A snack of shrimp, raw nuts, or slices of roast beef
Lunch:	Salad (large serving of lettuce, tomato, vinegar and oil dressing) Vegetables if desired Only ½ slice of bread or toast, with plenty of butter Beverage (herb tea or cereal coffee)
2 Hours before Dinner:	A light snack of raw nuts, cheese, or celery stuffed with cheese.
Dinner:	Soup if desired (not thickened with flour) Vegetables Liberal portion of meat, fish, or poultry Beverage (herb tea or cereal coffee)
Every 2 Hours until Bedtime:	A small handful of nuts or another desired protein.

NOTE: Baked potatoes or rice may at times be substituted for bread unless the condition is severe.

AVOID ABSOLUTELY:

Alcoholic and soft drinks such as club soda, dry ginger ale, whiskey and liquors

Sugar, candy, and other sweets such as cakes, pies, pastries, sweet custards, puddings, and ice cream

Caffeine - ordinary coffee, strongly brewed tea and beverages containing caffeine

Spaghetti, macaroni, noodles, donuts, jams, jellies, marmalades (starch and sugar)

Wines, cordials, cocktails, and beers (alcohol is high in carbohydrates)

Hydrogenated fats, partially hydrogenated fats, and fried foods

Allowable Oils: Butter, virgin olive oil, sesame oil, linseed oil (food grade, *not boiled*)

Four-Day Rotation Diet*

Day One

Food Families:

Citrus:	Lemon, orange, grapefruit, lime, tangerine, kumquat, citron
Banana:	Banana, plantain, arrowroot (musa)
Palm:	Coconut, date, date sugar
Parsley:	Carrots, parsnips, celery, celery seed, celeriac, anise, dill, fennel, cumin, parsley, coriander, caraway
Beet:	Beets, spinach, swiss chard, lamb's quarters (greens)
Pepper:	Black and white pepper, peppercorn
Herbs:	Nutmeg, mace
Cashew:	Cashew, pistachio, mango
Bird:	All fowl and game birds including chicken, turkey, duck, goose, guinea, pigeon, quail, pheasant, *eggs*
Tea:	Comfrey tea (Borage family), fennel tea
Oil:	Coconut oil, fats from any bird listed above, butter
Sweetener:	Use sparingly: Date sugar, orange honey (if honey is not used on another day of rotation), beet sugar
Juices:	Juices may be made and used without adding sweeteners from the following: Fruits: Any listed above in any combination Vegetables: Any listed above in any combination desired, including fresh comfrey
Grains:	Wheat
Fish:	Salmon, tuna

*Patients may wish to make their own rotation diets. The four-day diet presented here is given to show how it *can* be done. The basic requirement is that menus be prepared for four days so that a food on the menu on one day is not included on the menus of the three intervening days.

Day Two

Food Families

Grape:	All varieties of grapes, raisins
Pineapple:	(Juice pack, water pack, or fresh)
Rose:	Strawberry, raspberry, blackberry, dewberry, loganberry, young berry, boysenberry, rose hips
Melon:	(Gourd) Watermelon, cucumber, cantaloupe, pumpkin, squash, other melons; zucchini, acorn, pumpkin, or squash seeds
Mallow:	Okra, cottonseed
Pea:	(Legume) Peas, black-eyed peas, dry beans, green beans, carob, soy beans, lentils, licorice, peanut, alfalfa
Subucaya:	Brazil nuts
Flaxseed:	Flaxseed
Mollusks:	Abalone, snail, squid, clam, mussel, oyster, scallop
Crustaceans:	Crab, crayfish, lobster, prawn, shrimp
Tea:	Alfalfa tea, fenugreek
Oil:	Soybean oil, peanut oil, cottonseed oil, butter
Sweeteners:	(Use sparingly) Carob syrup
Clover honey:	If honey is not used on another day
Juices:	Juices may be made and used without added sweeteners from the following:
	Fruits or berries: Any listed above in any combination desired
	Vegetables: Any listed above in any combination desired including fresh alfalfa and some legumes
Fish:	Sardines, kippers, halibut
Grains:	Corn, millet
Red meat:	Beef, veal

Day Three

Food Families:

Apple:	Apple, pear, quince
Mulberry:	Mulberry, figs, breadfruit
Honeysuckle:	Elderberry
Olive:	Black or green or stuffed with pimento
Gooseberry:	Currant, gooseberry
Buckwheat:	Buckwheat
Aster:	Lettuce, chicory, endive, escarole, artichoke, dandelion, sunflower seeds, tarragon
Potato:	Potato, tomato, eggplant, peppers (red & green), chili pepper, paprika, cayenne, ground cherries
Lily (onion):	Onion, garlic, asparagus, chives, leeks
Spurge:	Tapioca
Herb:	Basil, savory, sage, oregano, horehound, catnip, spearmint, peppermint, thyme, marjoram, lemon balm
Walnut:	English walnut, black walnut, pecan, hickory nut, butternut
Pedalium:	Sesame
Beech:	Chestnut
Salt-water fish:	Sea herring, anchovy, cod, sea bass, sea trout, mackerel, swordfish, flounder, sole
Fresh-water fish:	Sturgeon, herring, whitefish, bass, perch
Tea:	Kaffir tea
Oil:	Safflower oil, butter
Honey:	(Use sparingly) Buckwheat, safflower, or sage honey (honey can be used if it has not been used any other day)
Juices:	Juices may be made and used without added sweeteners from the following: Fruits: Any listed above in any combination desired Vegetables and herbs: Any listed above in any combination desired
Red meat:	Lamb, mutton
Grains:	Rice, wild rice

Day Four

Food Families:

Plum:	Plum, cherry, peach, apricot, nectarine, almond, wild cherry
Blueberry:	Blueberry, huckleberry, cranberry, wintergreen
Pawpaw:	Pawpaw, papaya, papain
Mustard:	Mustard, turnip, radish, horseradish, watercress, cabbage, kraut, chinese cabbage, broccoli, cauliflower, brussel sprouts, collards, kale, kohlrabi, rutabaga
Laurel:	Avocado, cinnamon, bay leaf, sassafras, cassia buds or bark
Sweet potato:	Sweet potatoes or yams
Grass:	Oats, barley, rye, cane, sorghum, bamboo sprouts
Orchid:	Vanilla
Protea:	Macadamia nut
Birch:	Filberts, hazelnuts
Conifer:	Pine nut
Fungus:	Mushrooms and yeast (brewer's yeast, etc.)
Bovine:	Milk products—butter, cheese, yogurt, milk products, oleomargarine
Tea:	Sassafras tea or papaya leaf tea, lemon verbena tea
Oil:	Butter
Sweetener:	(Use sparingly) Cane, sugar, sorghum, molasses. Avocado honey if honey is not used on another day
Juices:	Juices may be made and used without added sweeteners, from the following: Fruits: Any listed above in any combination desired Vegetables: Any listed above in any combination desired, including any of the tea herbs, obtained fresh

Candida albicans Diet
(Strict yeast and mold avoidance list)

	Foods Permitted	Foods Omitted
Beverages:	Home-squeezed juice of peeled fruit, cow and goat milk, spring water, tap water	Alcohol, chocolate drinks, coffee (regular and decaffinated), sodas, tea (black and herbal), canned or frozen juices
Breads, cereals, grains:	*NO* grain products	*All* grain products are to be avoided
Diary products:	Butter, eggs, cow and goat milk, and plain yogurt	Cheeses, ice cream, margarine, flavored yogurt, sour cream, tofu, buttermilk
Fish and seafood:	Tuna in water, all other fish and seafood that is not breaded such as bass, bluefish, carp, clam, codfish, crab, flounder, haddock, halibut, herring, lobster, mackerel, oyster, pike, perch, swordfish, salmon, sardine, scallop, shrimp, smelt, trout, whitefish, etc.	Tuna in oil, breaded fish or seafood of any kind
Fruits:	Apple, avocado, banana, grapefruit, lemon-lime, nectarine, orange, peach, pear, pineapple, plum, tangerine. All fruit must be *fresh* and *peeled.* All fruit has yeast on its surface and should be peeled.	Blackberry, blueberry, cantaloupe, cherry, date, fig, grape, honeydew melon, prune, raspberry, raisin, strawberry, watermelon
Meats and poultry:	Beef, chicken, duck, lamb, beef liver, pork, turkey, veal	Fried or breaded meats, hot dogs, cold cuts, gravy

Candida albicans Diet (Continued)

	FOODS PERMITTED	FOODS OMITTED
Nuts:	None	All
Vegetables:	Beet, cabbage (peel off outer leaves), carrot, cucumber, eggplant, lettuce (peel off outer leaves), onion, parsnip, potato (sweet and white), pumpkin, radish, squash, tomato, turnip. All vegetables have yeast on the surface and should be peeled.	Artichoke, asparagus, broccoli, brussels sprouts, cauliflower, celery, corn, endive, green pepper kidney beans, kohlrabi, leek, lentil, lima beans, mushrooms, black olives, parsley, green peas, pimento, red pepper, rhubarb, soy beans, spinach, stringbeans
Miscellaneous:		Avoid monosodium glutamate and Accent seasonings, herbs, spices

Additional Information

Some individuals are unusually sensitive to yeasts and molds. For such persons, a trial diet which eliminates all foods and drinks that contain yeasts or molds is suggested.

Persons on this diet should keep a food and symptom diary for at least two or three weeks to help spot any changes and/or unsuspected infractions. In the beginning, the diet must be adhered to 100 percent. Then patients may be able to ease up on the diet and discover how strict they need to be to control symptoms.

All sugars and artificial colors, flavors, and preservatives are to be avoided on general grounds as well as to simplify the picture for this yeast/mold elimination diet.

ALWAYS READ LABELS CAREFULLY.

Most of the following items contain yeasts or molds:

1. All grains, such as wheat and corn, have small amounts of yeast or mold on their surfaces. Flours and cereals are often enriched with B vitamins that are usually derived from yeast. Also leavening or baker's yeast is often added to grain products. Breads, rolls, biscuits, buns, pretzels, crackers, cookies, cakes, and pies.

2. All nuts and seeds, dried fruits, teas (black and herbal), herbs, and spices (such as cinnamon and pepper) have yeast or mold on their surfaces.
3. Cheeses of all kinds, including cottage cheese, sour cream, tofu, and buttermilk contain mold. *Plain* yogurt is acceptable.
4. Yeast is present in all fermented beverages: all alcoholic beverages, medications containing alcohol and root beer and ginger ale.
5. Most condiments contain vinegar or other fermentation products: catsup, mayonnaise, salad dressings, barbeque sauce, tomato sauce, soy sauce, miso, tamari sauce, mincemeat, horseradish, sauerkraut, olives, and pickles.
6. Malt products contain some yeast: malted milk and some cereals and candies.
7. Mushrooms and truffles are mold foods.
8. Many vitamins contain or are derived from yeast. Check the labels and if in doubt, ask.
9. Antibiotics are often derived from mold cultures. If in doubt, ask.

APPENDIX II

The Clymer Health Clinic

The Clymer Health Clinic is a complete center for health and rehabilitation. Founded in 1969, with G. E. Poesnecker, N.D., D.C., as director, it continues the work in natural healing begun in the early decades of this century by the late R. Swinburne Clymer, M.D., one of America's giants in natural healing.

Staffed by disciples of Dr. Clymer's methods, the Clinic is a leader in holistic health care using naturally oriented techniques. Medical, chiropractic, classical homeopathic, naturopathic, and metabolic therapy services are provided. Adjunct therapies, such as nutritional testing and psychological counseling, are available. There are few health-stimulating techniques or diagnostic systems with which Clinic staff are unfamiliar. Those in daily use are the ones which have stood the test of time and have proven effective.

Each patient is considered individually at the Clymer Health Clinic, and treatment is tailored to the patient's condition and bodily balances. Because preventive care is stressed, many conditions are diagnosed and treated before they get a firm hold on a patient. Throughout treatment, emphasis is on nutritional counseling and education.

Since its founding, expansion of the Clinic has been continuous. At the pharmacy, a registered pharmacist dispenses remedies. A restaurant serves delicious, well-balanced meals. For patients from a distance or with health conditions that require frequent treatments or special diets, the guest house provides comfortable, relaxing accommodations.

The health and well-being of the patient is the prime consideration of all Clinic staff.

APPENDIX III:

Toxicities In Our Environment

Aluminum

The toxicity of aluminum has long been a disputed subject. Although many scientists did not previously consider aluminum to pose a significant health risk, recent evidence seriously questions this conclusion. Research now suggests that aluminum may interfere with normal body functioning at levels lower than previously assumed, and there have been increasing reports of aluminum toxicity from environmental exposure.

Sources. Aluminum cooking vessels, baking powder (aluminum sulfate), aluminum-containing antacids, deodorants and anti-perspirants, aluminum dust from industrial aluminum manufacturing, building construction materials, household and industrial utensils, insulated cables and wiring, packaging materials (*e.g.*, aluminum foil), fine aluminum powder used in bronze paint, aluminum cans, drinking water (alum used to kill bacteria), soil (naturally occurring ores), coal burning, plants including those used as food, beer, milk, and milk products (from equipment), alum used in food processing—pickles, maraschino cherries, medicinal aluminum compounds used externally to treat dermatitis, wounds, and burns, nasal spray (alum), toothpaste, ceramics (made from AI_2O_3 clay), dental amalgams, cigarette filters, tobacco smoke, automotive exhausts, pesticides, animal feed, FD&C color additives, vanilla powder, table salt and seasonings, bleached flour, American cheese, fumigant residues in foods (aluminum phosphide), Kaopectate and other medications containing kaolin (aluminum silicate), feldspar and mica, McIntyre aluminum powder (used in prophylaxis of silicosis), aluminum silicate paste (arthritis treatment), sutures with wound-healing coatings containing aluminum, aluminum chelates of polysaccharide-sulfuric acid esters for peptic ulcer treatment, aluminum nicotineate (hypercholesterolemia treatment).

Occupational Exposures. Manufacturing of aluminum abrasives, treating bauxite ore to obtain alumina, production of aluminum sulfate (alum) from bauxite ore, manufacturing of aluminum products, aluminum alloy manufacturing, paper industry, glass industry, textile industry (waterproofing), use of aluminum abrasives in many industrial operations, manufacturing of aluminum metal powders, synthetic leather manufacturing, aluminum welding, porcelain industry, explosives manufacturing, pyrotechnical devices manufacturing and use.

Signs and Symptoms. Aluminum pneumoconiosis (inhalation of Al dust): pneumothorax, pulmonary fibrosis with emphysema, dyspnea, right-sided cardiac hypertrophy, Shaver's disease: cough, substernal pain, weakness, fatigue, bilateral lace-like shadowing on lung X-ray; phosphate binding in gastrointestinal tract—aching muscles, rickets, osteoporosis; skin reactions (from Al antiperspirants), miliaria (acute inflammation of sweat glands); encephalopathy, senile dementia (Alzheimer's disease), nephritis, hypatic dysfunction, gastric distress, GI inflammation, flatulence, and acid eructation (belching), colitis, hyperactivity in children, psychosis in children.

Arsenic

Arsenic is a common environmental contaminant derived from natural and anthropogenic sources. Both oral ingestion and inhalation of arsenic are modes of intoxication. Arsenical toxicity is highly dependent on the chemical form, oxidation state, and route of exposure. Natural concentrations of arsenic in foodstuffs are usually rapidly absorbed, but also quickly excreted. Absorbed arsenic is transported by the blood to the kidneys, liver, spleen, skin, hair, and nails in that order. Some arsenic may remain in tissues long after it has disappeared from the blood, urine, and feces.

Sources. Rat poisons, insecticide residues on fruits and vegetables, herbicide residues on cottonseed products, wine (if arsenical insecticides used in vineyards), drinking water, well water, seafood, some kelp supplements, seawater, feed additives (poultry and livestock), coal burning, air polluted by arsenic dust from industrial plants, wood preservatives, wallpaper dye and plaster (containing volatile arsenicals), Paris green (arsenic containing pigment formerly used in ornaments, toys, curtains, carpets), some household detergents, colored chalk, automobile exhaust.

Occupational Exposures. Smelter workers, chemical workers handling inorganic arsenic, vintners working with arsenical insecticides, sheep dip workers using sodium arsenite, gold miners (associated arsenic ores), processors of taconite (low-grade iron ore), acetylene workers, alloy makers, aniline color workers, bleaching powder makers, boiler operators, bookbinders, bronze makers, colored-candle makers, canners, ceramic enamel workers, painters, paperhangers, petroleum refinery workers, plumbers, solderers, tree sprayers, wood preservative makers, hide preservers, taxidermists, weed sprayers, forestry workers.

Signs and Symptoms. Headache, drowsiness, confusion, brittle nails, follicular dermatitis, hoarse voice, Raynaud's phenomenon (poor circulation to extremities), weakness and muscular atrophy, palmar and plantar keratoses, pigmented spots on trunk, atypical (precancerous) keratoses on hands, feet, and trunk, squamous cell carcinoma of skin, "Mees lines" (transverse white ridges or parallel lines on nails), erythromelalgia (burning pain, redness, swelling of hands and feet), hemiplegia, sensory changes (parathesias, hyperesthesias, neuralgias, myalgia), garlic odor on breath and perspiration, goiter, heart failure, hypertension, hepatomegaly and jaundice.

Cadmium

Cadmium is toxic to every bodily system whether ingested, injected, or inhaled and tends to accumulate in body tissues. Consequently, there is concern about the increase in environmental cadmium that has occurred as a result of its increasing industrial use. Inhaled cadmium is usually better absorbed than ingested cadmium. Once absorbed, the elimination rate is generally very slow. The toxicity of cadmium, however, is significantly influenced by dietary intake of other elements such as zinc, copper, and selenium.

Sources. Drinking water, soft water, causing uptake of Cd from galvanized pipes, soft drinks from vending machines with Cd piping, refined wheat flour (increased Cd:Zn ration), evaporated milk, many processed foods, oysters, kidney, liver, rice (irrigated by Cd-contaminated water), soil, cigarette smoke, tobacco, superphosphate fertilizers, Cadmium alloys (e.g., dental prosthetics), ceramics, paint pigments, electroplating, cadmium-vapor lamps, tools rustproofed with cadmium, marine hardware rustproofed with cadmium, welding metal, solders, silver polish, polyvinyl plastics, fungicides, pesticides, sewage sludge and effluents, copper refineries, dust in urban streets, homes, businesses, and schools, rubber carpet backing, wear of rubber tires, burning of motor oil, plastic tapes, black polyethylene, black rubber, nickel-cadmium battery manufacturing, zinc or polymetallic ore smelting, paint manufacture using cadmium pigments, painting with cadmium pigments, jewelry making, cadmium alloy manufacturing, ceramic making using cadmium, electroplating metals with cadmium, process engraving, cadmium vapor lamp manufacturing, rustproofing tools, marine hardware, soldering, tetraethyl lead manufacturing (uses diethyl cadmium), fungicide manufacturing.

Signs and Symptoms. Fatigue, hypertension (possibly related to increased concentration of Cd in renal parenchyma), iron-deficiency anemia, emphysema, Itai-Itai (osteomalacia in parous women over forty years of age with dietary deficiencies), slight liver damage, anosmia (loss of sense of smell), yellow coloring of teeth, reduced birthweight in newborns, renal colic (with passage of calculi), nephrocalcinosis, hypercalcuria, pain in lower back and legs, pain in sternum, "Milkman's syndrome" (lines of pseudofracture in scapula, femur, ileum), hypophosphatemia, possible rheumatoid arthritis, decreased production of active vitamin D, decreased pulmonary function, proteinuria, glucosuria, and aminoaciduria (following nine years of inhaling Cd oxide), possible prostatic cancer (in workers exposed to Cd oxide), possible carcinogenesis, increased mortality.

Copper

Although copper is an essential element, there are situations in which the possibility of human copper toxicity requires consideration. Wilson's disease (an inborn error of human metabolism) represents a special case of copper toxicosis. Large amounts of copper accumulate in the liver, kidney, and brain of those with this disease. Copper can be absorbed by the lungs, skin, uterus, and gastrointestinal tract. The toxic effects of copper are related to the adequacy of other elements, such as zinc.

Sources. Drinking water, copper plumbing and piping, surface and ground water, animal and industrial waste, fungicides and insecticides, sewage sludge, oysters, liver, nuts, and chocolate, vinegar, carbonated beverages, or citrus juices if prolonged contact with copper, beer (from copper piping and brew kettles), refrigerator ice makers, hemodialysis, copper intrauterine contraceptive devices (IUDs), copper in dental prostheses, milk (accumulates copper from heated copper rollers during pasteurization), industrial emissions, swimming pools (fungicide), copper cookware, vitamin-mineral supplements.

Signs and Symptoms. Accidental poisoning (acute): vomiting, diarrhea, jaundice, impaired liver function, hemoglobinuria, hematuria, oliguria, hypotension, coma, death; copper metal fume fever: chills, fever, aching muscles, dryness of mouth and throat, headache, digestive disorders; arthritis, scleroderma, eczema, schizophrenia, postpartum psychosis, autism, gingivitis (caused by Cu-containing dental work), nasal irritation, bitter taste, anemia (iron deficiency), atherosclerosis.

Lead

Lead has long been known as a toxic element. At one time it was believed that the only significant sources of increased lead ingestion were plaster, paint, or industrial exposure. Although this is probably true for acute lead poisoning, it is not true for chronic lead toxicity. The increasing prevalence of lead as an environmental contaminant has led to subclinical exposures which often result in subtle, yet significant, adverse health effects. Lead may enter the body through ingestion, inhalation, or skin eruption. Adults normally absorb 5 to 10 percent of ingested lead, while children may readily absorb up to 50 percent. Inhaled lead is absorbed at 25 - 100 percent, depending on the lead particle size. Tolerance to lead varies with age, form, and source of the lead and with the composition of the diet being consumed.

Source. Atmospheric lead—motor vehicle exhausts, lead smelters, coal burning, refining lead scrap, burning materials containing lead; dust and dirt, leaded house paint, drinking water, lead plumbing, vegetation growing by roadside, vegetables grown in lead-contaminated soils, canned fruit and fruit juice, canned evaporated milk, milk from animals grazing on Pb-contaminated pastures, bone meal, organ meats, especially liver, lead-arsenate pesticides, wine (leaded caps), rainwater, snow, improperly glazed pottery, painted glassware, pencils (paint), toothpaste, newsprint, colored printed materials, spitballs, eating utensils, curtain weights, putty, car batteries, cigarette ash, tobacco, lead shot, mascara, painted children's toys, PVC containers, canned pet food, hair dyes (progressive darkeners).

Occupational Exposures. Acid finishers, actors, battery makers, blacksmiths, bookbinders, bottle cap makers, brass founders, brass polishers, braziers, brick burners, brick makers, bronzers, brush-makers, cable makers, cable splicers, canners, cartridge makers, chemical equipment makers, chlorinated paraffin makers, chippers, cigar makers, crop dusters, cutlery makers, decorators (pottery), demolition workers, dental technicians, diamond polishers, dye makers, dyers, electronic device makers, electroplaters, electrotypers, embroidery workers, emery wheel makers, enamel burners, enamelers, enamel makers, explosives makers, farmers, file cutters, firemen, flower makers (artificial), foundry workers, galvanizers, garage mechanics, glass makers, glass polishers, gold refiners, gun barrel browners, incandescent lamp makers, ink makers, insecticide makers, insecticide users, Japan makers, Janers, jewellers, junk metal refiners, kiln workers, labelers (paint can), lacquer makers, lead burners, lead counterweight makers, lead flooring makers, lead foil makers, lead mill workers, lead miners, lead pipe makers, lead salt makers, lead shield makers, lead smelters, lead stearate makers, lead workers, linoleum makers, linotypists, linseed oil boilers, lithotransfer workers, match makers, metal burners, metal cutters, metal grinders, metal polishers, metal refiners, metal refinishers, metallizers, mirror silverers, musical instrument makers, nitric acid workers, nitroglycerin makers, painters, paint makers, paint pigment makers, paperhangers, patent leather makers, pearl makers (imitation), pharmaceutical makers, photography workers, pipe fitters, plastic workers, plumbers, printers, policemen, pottery glaze mixers, pottery workers, putty makers, pyroxylin-plastic workers, riveters, roofers, rubber buffers, rubber makers, rubber reclaimers, scrap metal workers, semi-conductor workers, service station attendants, sheet metal workers, shellac makers, ship dismantlers, shoe stainers, shot makers, silk weighters, slushers (porcelain enameling), solderers, solder makers, steel engravers, stereotypists, tannery workers, television picture tube makers, temperers, textile makers, tile makers, tinners, type founders, typesetters, vanadium compound makers, varnish makers, vehicle tunnel attendants, wallpaper printers, welders, wood stainers, zinc mill workers, zinc smelter chargers.

Common Nonoccupational Lead Exposures. Ceramics, pottery, and related hobbies, stained glass work, electronics and related hobbies involving extensive soldering, firing ranges, hunting (especially those who cast their own bullets), eating or drinking (from improperly fired lead-glazed ceramic tableware), eating lead-bearing paint, burning battery casings, consuming illicitly distilled whiskey, extensive auto driving (especially in cities), extensive work with motor fuels, painting with lead-containing paints, home plumbing repairs (lead pipe systems), exterminating.

Signs and Symptoms. Headache, depression, insomnia and/or drowsiness, fatigue, nervousness, irritability, dizziness, confusion and disorientation, anxiety, muscle weakness and wasting, saturnine gout, aching muscles and bones, abdominal pain, loss of appetite, loss of weight, constipation, hypertension, kidney function defects, reproductive defects—decreased fertility in men or spontaneous abortion in women, adrenal gland function impaired, iron-deficiency anemia, blue-black lead lines near base of teeth.

Symptoms More Common in Children. Hyperactivity, temper tantrums, withdrawal, frequent crying for no apparent reason, fearfulness, refusal to play, other emotional or behavioral problems, drowsiness, learning disabilities, speech disturbances, perceptual motor dysfunctions, mental retardation, seizures or convulsions, ataxia, encephalopathy.

Mercury

Mercury, long known as a toxic element, has evoked increasing concern in recent years because of its increasing use in industry and agriculture and the burning of fossil fuels. Methylmercury compounds and elemental mercury vapor are the two forms most likely to be involved in human exposures. In addition, the conversion of elemental mercury and mercury compounds by bacteria to the more toxic methylmercury also poses potential threats to human health. Ingested methylmercury is readily absorbed through the gastrointestinal tract and inhaled mercury vapor is easily retained by the pulmonary system. Skin absorption of mercury may also occur.

Sources: Mercury-silver amalgam (dental fillings), broken thermometers and barometers, consumption of grain seeds treated with methylmercury fungicide, fish and marine mammals, mercuric chloride (used in histology laboratories), calomel (body powders and talcs), mercury-containing cosmetics, latex and solvent-thinned paints, organic mercurials (diuretics), air polluted by industrial mercury vapor, mercury-polluted industrial water, clothing worn by mercury workers, hemorrhoid suppositories using mercurials, Mercurochrome and Merthiolate (thimerosal), fabric softeners, floor waxes and polishes, air conditioner filters, wood preservatives, cinnabar (used in jewelry), batteries with mercury cells, fungicides for use on lawns, trees, shrubs, and so on, tanning leather, felt, adhesives, laxatives (containing calomel), skin-lightening creams, psoriatic ointments, photoengraving, tatooing, laboratory and industrial equipment using metallic mercury, sewage sludge used as fertilizer contaminates soil, sewage disposal (may release thousands of tons of Hg annually world wide).

Occupational Exposures. Amalgam makers, bactericide makers, barometer makers, mercury battery makers, boilermakers, bronzers, calibration instrument makers, percussion cap loaders, carbon brush makers, caustic soda makers, ceramic workers, chlorine makers, dental amalgam makers, dentists, direct current meter workers, disinfectant makers, disinfectors, drug makers, dye makers, electric apparatus makers, electroplaters, embalmers, explosives makers, farmers, fingerprint detectors, fireworks makers, fish cannery workers, fungicide makers, fur preservers, fur processors, gold extractors, histology technicians, ink makers, insecticide makers, investment casting workers, jewelers, chemical laboratory workers, fluorescent lampmakers, Manometer makers, mercury workers, mercury miners, mirror makers, neon light makers, paintmakers, papermakers, percussion cap makers, pesticide workers, photographers, pressure gauge makers, mercury refiners, seed handlers, silver extractors, mercury switch makers, tannery workers, taxidermists, textile printers, thermometer makers, vinyl chloride manufacturers, wood preservative workers.

Signs and Symptoms. Elemental mercury vapor exposure: insomnia, shyness, nervousness, dizziness, loss of memory, lack of self-control, irritability, anxiety, loss of self-confidence, drowsiness, depression, loss of weight, loss of appetite, tremors; severe cases: hallucinations, manic depression; organic mercury exposure: earliest symptoms—fatigue, headache, forgetfulness; later findings—numbness and tingling of the lips and feet, muscle weakness progressing to paralysis, loss of vision, hearing difficulty, speech disorders, loss of memory, incoordination, emotional instability, dermatitis, renal damage, general brain dysfunctions; late symptoms—coma, death.

Nickel

Nickel can be a toxic element in man. It can interact by four routes of entry into the body. These are oral ingestion, inhalation, parenteral administration, and percutaneous absorption. Nickel or nickel salts are relatively nontoxic when taken orally. Nickel toxicity from parenteral administration has only been observed experimentally. Percutaneous absorption may manifest as nickel dermatitis and is relatively common. The inhalation of nickel carbonyl causes the most serious type of nickel toxicity, although it usually occurs only in occupational workers due to an industrial accident.

Sources. Stainless steel cookware (Ni taken up by acid foods), tobacco smoke, contamination of air, drinking water, soil, and vegetation by industrial nickel, testing of nuclear devices (radionuclide Ni-63), exhausts of automobiles and trucks, burning of coal and oil for power generation, burning of fuel oil for space heating, wear of automobile tires and brake linings, superphosphate fertilizers, dissolved nickel from food-processing equipment, hydrogenated fats and oils, baking powder, nickel-cadmium storage batteries.

Sources of Contact for Allergic Individuals. Nickel jewelry, nickel coins, clothing fasteners, tools, cooking utensils, stainless steel kitchens, detergents, prostheses, medical appliances, metal chairs, thimbles, needles, scissors, zippers, bobby pins, fountain pens.

Occupational Exposures. Nickel mining, nickel refining, nickel electroplating, nickel alloy makers, nickel-cadmium battery workers, chemical industry, electronics and computer industry, food processing, nickel waste disposal and recycling, ceramics industry workers, duplicating machine workers, dyers, ink makers, jewelers, spark plug makers, rubber workers, plastics industry, coin manufacturers, automotive parts makers.

Signs and Symptoms. Nickel dermatitis ("nickel itch") is manifested by itching or burning causing a papular erythema of the web of the fingers, wrist, and forearms. The reaction is largely allergic in nature. Acute toxicity from inhalation of nickel carbonyl: dyspnea, tachypnea, headache, insomnia, fever, cyanosis, apathy, anorexia, vomiting, diarrhea. Pulmonary cancer (from nickel in tobacco smoke).

References

Preface

1. Poesnecker, G.E. *It's Only Natural.* Quakertown, Pa., G.E. Poesnecker, 1975. (3rd ed., 1981)

Chapter I: The Nature of the Disease

1. Sajous, Charles E. de M. *The Internal Secretions and the Practice of Medicine.* Philadelphia, F. A. Davis Company, 1903. (10th ed., 1922)
2. Harrower, Henry R. *Practical Organic Therapy, the Internal Secretions in General Practice,* 3d ed. Glendale, Calif., The Harrower Laboratory, 1922.
3. Tintera, John W. The hypoadrenocortical state and its management. *New York State Journal of Medicine* 55:1869, 1955.
4. Tintera, John W. Stabilizing homeostasis in the recovered alcoholic through endocrine therapy: Evaluation of the hypoglycemic factor. *Journal of the American Geriatrics Society* 6:126, 1966.
5. Polonsky, Kenneth, and others. Relation of counterregulatory responses to hypoglycemia in type I diabetes. *New England Journal of Medicine* 307 (18):1106-1112, October 28, 1982.
6. Tintera, John W. What you should know about your glands and allergies. *Women's Day* February 1959, pp. 28-29, 92.
7. Rapoport, M. I., and Beisel, W. R. Inter-relations between adrenocortical functions and infectious illness. *New England Journal of Medicine* 280(10):541-546, May 6, 1969.
8. Prange, A.J., and others. Effects of thyrotropin-releasing hormone in depression. *Lancet* 2:999-1002, 1972.
9. Loosen, Peter T., and Prange, Arthur J., Jr. Serum thryotropin response to thyrotropin-releasing hormone in psychiatric patients: A review. *American Journal of Psychiatry* 139(4):405-416, April 1982.
10. Gold, Mark S., and others. Grades of thyroid failure in 100 depressed and anergic psychiatric inpatients. *American Journal of Psychiatry* 138(2):253-255, February 1981.
11. Gold, Mark S., and others. Hypothyroidism and depression: Evidence from complete thyroid function evaluation. *Journal of the American Medical Association* 245(19):1919-1922, May 15, 1981.
12. Amsterdam, Jay, and others. Thyrotropin-releasing hormone's mood-elevating effects in depressed patients, anorectic patients, and normal volunteers. *American Journal of Psychiatry* 138(1):115-118, January 1981.
13. Selye, Hans. General adaptation syndrome and diseases of adaptation. *Journal of Clinical Endocrinology and Metabolism* 6:117-230, 1946.
14. Selye, Hans. *The Stress of Life.* New York, McGraw-Hill Book Company, Inc., 1956.

Chapter II: The Nature of the Patient

1. Poesnecker, G.E. *It's Only Natural.* Quakertown, Pa., G.E. Poesnecker, 1975. (3d ed., 1981)

Chapter III: Clinical Treatment

1. Harrower, Henry. *Practical Organic Therapy, the Internal Secretions in General Practice,* 3d ed. Glendale Calif., The Harrower Library, 1922.
2. Poesnecker, G.E. *It's Only Natural.* Quakertown, Pa., G. E. Poesnecker, 1975. (3d ed., 1981)
3. Franklin, Benjamin. *Autobiography.* New York, The Macmillan Company, 1901.

Chapter V: Patient and Family Responsibilities

1. Poesnecker, G.E. *It's Only Natural.* Quakertown, Pa., G.E. Poesnecker, 1975. (3d ed., 1981)

Chapter VI: Sex and the Adrenal Syndrome Patient

1. Poesnecker, G. E. *Creative Sex.* Quakertown, Pa., Clymer Health Clinic, 1976.
2. Pfeiffer, Carl C., and the Publications Committee of the Brain Bio Center. *Mental and Elemental Nutrients.* New Canaan, Conn., Keats Publishing, Inc., 1975. Chapter 48.
3. Ambrus, J. L., and others. Progestational agents and blood coagulation. VII. Thromboembolic and other complications of oral contraceptive therapy—relationship to pretreatment levels of blood coagulation factors. Summary report of a 10-year study. *American Journal of Obstetrics and Gynecology* 125:1057-1062, August 15, 1976.
4. Beral, V., and others. The pill and circulatory disease. *American Heart Journal* 97:263-264, February 1979.
5. Zakin, D., and others. Complete and partial uterine perforation and embedding following insertion of uterine devices. II. Diagnostic methods, prevention and management. *Obstetrics and Gynecology Survey* 36:401-412, August 1981.
6. Connell, E. B. Side effects of IUDs. *International Journal of Gynaecology* 15(2):153-156, 1977.
7. Burkman, R., and others. Relationship of genital tract actinomycetes and the development of pelvic inflammatory disease. *American Journal of Obstetrics and Gynecology* 143:585-589, July 1, 1982.
8. Drew, N. C. Genital and pelvic actinomycosis. Case report. *British Journal of Obstetrics and Gynaecology* 88(7):776-777, July 1981.
9. Gupta, P. K., and others. Actinomycetes and the IUD: An update. *Acta Cytology (Baltimore)* 22:281-282, September-October 1978.
10. Clark, Blake. Your emotions can make you ill. *Reader's Digest* 100:129-132, May 1972.
11. Jonas, Gerald. Manfred Clynes and the science of sentics. *Saturday Review* 55:42-46, May 13, 1972.

Chapter VII: Stresses of the Environment — Internal and External

1. Sajous, Charles E. de M. *The Internal Secretions and the Practice of Medicine.* Philadelphia, F. A. Davis Company, 1903. (10th ed., 1922).
2. Poesnecker, G. E. *It's Only Natural.* Quakertown, Pa., G. E. Poesnecker, 1975. (3d ed., 1981).
3. Wuerthele-Caspe, Virginia, and others. Cultural properties and pathogenecity of certain microorganisms obtained from various proliferative and neoplastic diseases. *American Journal of Medical Science* 220:638-648, December 1950.

4. Wuerthele-Caspe, Virginia, and others. Intracellular acid-fast micro-organism. *Journal of American Medical Women's Association* 11(4):120-129, April 1956.
5. Livingston, Virginia Wuerthele-Caspe, and Livingston, Afton Munck. Some cultural, immunological and biochemical properties of *Progenitor cryptocides. Transactions of the New York Academy of Science,* Series II 36(6):569-582, June 1974.
6. Livingston, Virginia Wuerthele-Caspe, and Livingston, Afton Munk. Demonstration of *Progenitor cryptocides* in the blood of patients with collagen and neoplastic diseases. *Transactions of the New York Academy of Science* 34(5):433-453, 1972.
7. Livingston, Virginia Wuerthele-Caspe, and Livingston, Afton Munk. A specific type of organism cultivated from malignancy: Bacteriology and proposed classification. *Annals of the New York Academy of Science* 174:636-654, October 30, 1970.
8. Truss, C. Orian. Restoration of immunologic competence to *Candida albicans. Journal of Orthomolecular Psychiatry* 9(4):287-301, 1980.
9. Truss, C. Orian. Role of *Candida albicans* in human illness. *Journal of Orthomolecular Psychiatry* 10(4):228, 1981.
10. Truss, C. Orian. Tissue injury induced by *Candida albicans. Journal of Orthomolecular Psychiatry* 7(1):17-37, 1978.
11. Loose, D. S., Schurman, D.J., and Feldman, David. *Nature* 293:477, 1981.
12. Feldman, David, and others. An estrogen-binding protein and endogenous ligand in Saccharomyces cerevisial: Possible hormone receptor system. *Science* 218:297-298, October 15, 1982.
13. Poesnecker, G.E. *Creative Sex.* Quakertown, Pa., Clymer Health Clinic, 1976.
14. Griffith, R. S., and others. Relation of arginine-lysine antagonism to herpes simplex growth in tissue culture. *Chemotherapy* 27(3):209-213, 1981.
15. Lysine prophylaxis in recurrent herpes simplex tabialis: A double-blind, controlled crossover study. *Acta Dermato-Venereologica (Stockholm)* 60(1):85-87, 1980.
16. Black, A. P. A new diagnostic method in allergic disease. *Pediatrics.* 17:5, 1956.
17. Bryan, William, and others. The application of in vitro cytotoxic reactions to clinical diagnosis of food allergy. In *Clinical Ecology,* edited by Lawrence D. Dickey. Springfield, Ill., Charles C Thomas, 1976.
18. Sheinkin, David, and others. Cytotoxic testing and characteristics of cytotoxic testing. In *The Food Connection.* Indianapolis, The Bobbs/Merrill Company, Inc., 1979, pp. 83-88.
19. Tintera, John W. The hypoadrenocortical state and its management. *New York State Journal of Medicine* 55:1869, 1955.
20. Tintera, John W. What you should know about your glands and allergies. *Woman's Day* February 1959, pp. 28-29, 92.
21. Dingle, Donald L. The cytotoxic microscope test. *Digest of Chiropractic Economics,* 23(3):70-71, Nov-Dec 1980.
22. Lehman, Carl W. The leukocytic food allergy test: A study of its reliability and reproducibility: Effect of diet and sublingual food drops on this test. *Annals of Allergy* 45:150-158, September 1980.
23. Grieco, Michael H. Controversial practices in allergy. *Journal of the American Medical Association* 247(22):3106-3111, June 11, 1982.
24. Boyles, John H., Jr. The validity of using the cytotoxic food test in clinical allergy, *Ear, Nose, and Throat Journal* 56(4):168-173, April 1977.
25. Ulett, G. A., and Perry, S. G. Cytotoxic testing and leukocyte increase as an index to food sensitivity. *Annals of Allergy* 33:23-32, January 1974.

26. Ulett, G. A., and Perry, S. G. Cytotoxic testing and leukocyte increase as an index to food sensitivity. II. Coffee and tobacco. *Annals of Allergy* 34:150-159, March 1975.
27. Philpott, William Henry. Ecologic, orthomolecular and behavioral contributions to psychiatry. *Journal of Orthomolecular Psychiatry* 3(4):356-370, 1974. (See especially pp. 359-360.)
28. Philpott, William Henry. Four-day rotation diet. In *Clinical Ecology*, edited by Lawrence D. Dickey. Springfield, Ill., Charles C Thomas 1976.
29. Mandell, Marshall, *Cerebral Reactions in Allergic Patients.* Presented at the 24th Annual Congress, American College of Allergists, Section on Neurologic Allergy, Washington, D. C., April 18, 1969.
30. Mandell, Marshall, and Scanlon, L. W. *Dr. Mandell's 5-Day Allergy Relief System.* New York, Thomas Y. Crowell Co., 1979.
31. Berg, Torsten L. O., and Johansson, S. G. O. Allergy diagnosis with the Radioallergosorbent Test. *Journal of Allergy and Clinical Immunology* 54(4):209-221, October 1974.
32. Merrett, T. G., and Merrett, J. The RAST principle and the use of mixed-allergen RAST as a screening test for IgE-mediated allergies. *Methods in Enzymology* 70(A):376-387, 1980.
33. Kaslow, Arthur L., and Miles, Richard B. *You Can Achieve Freedom from Chronic Disease.* Los Angeles. J. P. Tarcher, Inc., 1979.
34. Pope, T., Jr., and Hughes, L. A. Pulsating irrigation: A simple, safe, effective treatment of many nasal complaints, *O.R.L. Digest* 36:10-12, August 1974.
35. Passwater, Richard. *Supernutrition for Healthy Hearts.* New York, The Dial Press, 1977, p. 112-118.
36. Pfeiffer, Carl C., and the Publications Committee of the Brain Bio Center. *Mental and Elemental Nutrients.* New Canaan, Conn., Keats Publishing, Inc., 1975.
37. Painter, Marylyn. Fluorescent lights and hyperactivity in children. An experiment. *Education Digest* 42:36-37, April 1977.
38. Ponte, L. How artificial light affects your health. *Reader's Digest* 118:131-134, February 1981.
39. Wurtman, Richard J. Effects of light on the human body *Scientific American* 233:68-77, July 1975.
40. Barnes, Broda O., and Galton, Lawrence. *Hypothyroidism. The Unsuspected Illness.* New York, Thomas Y. Crowell Co., 1976.
41. McCabe, Donald Lee. Kryptopyrrole in clinic practice. *Osteopathic Medicine* September 1980, pages 43-59.
42. Sauberlich, H. E., and others. *Laboratory Tests for the Assessment of Nutritional Status.* Boca Raton, Fla., CRC Press, Inc., 1979.

VIII: A Final Word

1. Buttram. Harold E., and Hoffman, John Chriss. *Vaccinations and Immune Malfunction.* Quakertown, Pa., Humanitarian Publishing Co., 1982.

INDEX